Orthoplastic Techniques for Lower Extremity Reconstruction — Part I

Editors

EDGARDO R. RODRIGUEZ-COLLAZO
SUHAIL MASADEH

CLINICS IN PODIATRIC MEDICINE AND SURGERY

www.podiatric.theclinics.com

Consulting Editor
THOMAS J. CHANG

October 2020 • Volume 37 • Number 4

ELSEVIER

1600 John F. Kennedy Boulevard • Suite 1800 • Philadelphia, Pennsylvania, 19103-2899

http://www.theclinics.com

CLINICS IN PODIATRIC MEDICINE AND SURGERY Volume 37, Number 4
October 2020 ISSN 0891-8422, ISBN-13: 978-0-323-76287-8

Editor: Lauren Boyle
Developmental Editor: Nicole Congleton

Clinics in Podiatric Medicine and Surgery (ISSN 0891-8422) is published quarterly by Elsevier Inc., 360 Park Avenue South, New York, NY 10010-1710. Months of issue are January, April, July, and October. Business and Editorial Offices: 1600 John F. Kennedy Blvd., Ste. 1800, Philadelphia, PA 19103-2899. Customer Service Office: 3251 Riverport Lane, Maryland Heights, MO 63043. Periodicals postage paid at New York, NY and additional mailing offices. Subscription prices are $304.00 per year for US individuals, $597.00 per year for US institutions, $100.00 per year for US students and residents, $382.00 per year for Canadian individuals, $721.00 for Canadian institutions, $457.00 for international individuals, $721.00 per year for international institutions, $100.00 per year for Canadian students/residents, and $220.00 per year for foreign students/residents. To receive student/resident rate, orders must be accompanied by name of affiliated institution, date of term, and the *signature* of program/residency coordinator on institution letterhead. Orders will be billed at individual rate until proof of status is received. Foreign air speed delivery is included in all *Clinics* subscription prices. All prices are subject to change without notice. POSTMASTER: Send address changes to *Clinics in Podiatric Medicine and Surgery*, Elsevier Health Sciences Division, Subscription Customer Service, 3251 Riverport Lane, Maryland Heights, MO 63043. **Customer Service: 1-800-654-2452 (US). From outside of the US, call 314-447-8871. Fax: 314-447-8029. E-mail: JournalsCustomerService-usa@elsevier.com (for print support); JournalsOnlineSupport-usa@elsevier.com (for online support).**

Reprints. For copies of 100 or more of articles in this publication, please contact the Commercial Reprints Department, Elsevier Inc., 360 Park Avenue South, New York, NY 10010-1710. Tel.: 212-633-3874; Fax: 212-633-3820; E-mail: reprints@elsevier.com.

Clinics in Podiatric Medicine and Surgery is covered in *MEDLINE/PubMed (Index Medicus)* and *EMBASE/Excerpta Medica*.

Printed in the United States of America.

Contributors

CONSULTING EDITOR

THOMAS J. CHANG, DPM
Clinical Professor and Past Chairman, Department of Podiatric Surgery, California College of Podiatric Medicine, Faculty, The Podiatry Institute, Redwood Orthopedic Surgery Associates, Santa Rosa, California, USA

EDITORS

EDGARDO R. RODRIGUEZ-COLLAZO, DPM
Department of Surgery, AMITA Health–St. Joseph Hospital, Fellowship Director, Complex Deformity Correction & Microsurgical Limb Reconstruction, Chicago, Illinois, USA

SUHAIL MASADEH, DPM
Associate Professor of Surgery, Director of Podiatric Surgery Residency, University of Cincinnati Medical Center, Chief of Surgical Podiatry, Cincinnati Veteran Affairs Medical Center, Cincinnati, Ohio, USA

AUTHORS

SHARIF R. ABDELFATTAH, DPM
Chief Resident, East Liverpool City Hospital, East Liverpool, Ohio, USA; Foot and Ankle Surgeon, Sullivan County Community Hospital, Sullivan, Indiana, USA

MOHAMED ABDEL-HAMID ROMEIH, MD
Assistant Professor of Orthopedic Surgery and Traumatology, Department of Orthopedic Surgery, Faculty of Medicine, Tanta University, Tanta University Hospital, Tanta, Egypt

CHRISTOPHER BIBBO, DO, DPM, FACS, FAAOS, FACFAS
Chief, Foot and Ankle Surgery, Plastic Reconstructive and Microsurgery and Limb Salvage, Orthopaedic Trauma, and Musculoskeletal Infection Services, Rubin Institute for Advanced Orthopedics, International Center for Limb Lengthening, Sinai Hospital of Baltimore, Baltimore, Maryland, USA

PHUOC V. BUI, DPM
Resident PGY-3, Department of Podiatric Surgery, TriHealth – Bethesda North Hospital, Montgomery, Ohio, USA

MATHEW CERNIGLIA, DPM, FACFAS, FAENS
Private Practice, Saginaw, Texas, USA

HASSAN CHAHADEH, MD
Chairman, Vision Park of Surgery Center, Shenandoah, Texas, USA

GRACE CHUANG CRAIG, DPM
Elevate Foot and Ankle, Rocky River, Ohio, USA

PETER A. CRISOLOGO, DPM
Assistant Professor, Department of Surgery, Division of Podiatric Surgery, University of Cincinnati Medical Center, Cincinnati, Ohio, USA

JOSE ANTONIO DELGADO PEREZ, MD
Pediatric Orthopedic Surgeon, Medical Staff of Pediatric Orthopedics, National Institute of Pediatrics, Mexico City, Mexico

ALEC J. DIERKSHEIDE, DPM
Resident, Department of Surgery, Division of Podiatric Surgery, University of Cincinnati Medical Center, Cincinnati, Ohio, USA

MOHAMED A. ELLABBAN, MD, MBBCh, MSc, MRCS
Assistant Professor of Plastic and Reconstructive Surgery, Suez Canal University Hospitals and Medical School, Ismailia, Egypt

MAHMOUD EL-ROSASY, MD
Professor of Orthopedic Surgery and Traumatology, Limb Lengthening and Reconstruction and Pediatric Orthopedics, Department of Orthopedic Surgery, Tanta University Hospital, Faculty of Medicine, Tanta University, Tanta, Egypt

MOHAMED FADEL, MD
Professor, Orthopedic and Trauma Surgery, Minia University Hospital, Minia, Egypt

RAMY X. FAHIM, DPM
Section Chief, Foot and Ankle Surgery, Mercy Health, Youngstown, Ohio, USA; Foot and Ankle Surgeon, Northern Ohio Medical Specialties (NOMS) Healthcare, Sandusky, Ohio, USA

AHMED ASHRAF FISAL, MSc
Assistant Lecturer of Orthopedic Surgery and Traumatology, Department of Orthopedic Surgery, Faculty of Medicine, Tanta University, Tanta University Hospital, Tanta, Egypt

CHRIS GREEN, DPM
Lower Extremity Reconstructive and Salvage Surgeon Fellow, American College of Foot and Ankle Surgeons, Medical Director, Integris Limb Salvage Center, Oklahoma City, Oklahoma, USA

JORDAN A. HENNING, DPM
Assistant Professor of Surgery, University of Cincinnati Medical Center, Staff Podiatrist, Cincinnati VA Medical Center, Cincinnati, Ohio, USA

LANCE JOHNSON, DPM
Resident Physician, University of Cincinnati Medical Center, Cincinnati, Ohio, USA

ARSHAD A. KHAN, DPM, FACFAS, FACFAOM
Volunteer Assistant Clinical Professor, Department of Orthopedic Surgery, Indiana University School of Medicine, Gary/Northwest, Indianapolis, Indiana, USA; Clinical Director, SpineTech Neurosurgeons, SpineTech Brain and Spine of South East Texas, Shenandoah, Texas, USA

ISRA M. KHAN, MD
Research Associate, Chicago Foot and Ankle Deformity Correction Center, Chicago, Illinois, USA; Shenandoah, Texas, USA

MOHAMED LAKLOUK, MD
Professor of Orthopedic Surgery, Faculty of Medicine, Minia University, Minia, Egypt

MICHAEL D. LIETTE, DPM
Resident Podiatric Physician, University of Cincinnati Medical Center, Cincinnati, Ohio, USA

ERWIN LO, MD
Clinical Assistant Professor, University of Texas Medical Branch, Mischer Neuroscience Institute, Houston, Texas, USA; Neurosurgeon and Founder of SpineTech, Brain and Spine Center of Southeast Texas, Beaumont, Texas, USA

SUHAIL MASADEH, DPM
Associate Professor of Surgery, Director of Podiatric Surgery Residency, University of Cincinnati Medical Center, Chief of Surgical Podiatry, Cincinnati Veteran Affairs Medical Center, Cincinnati, Ohio, USA

PHI P. NGUYEN, MD
Associate Professor of Surgery, McGowan Medical School, Medical Director, MIA Plastic Surgery, Medical Director, MILA Med Spa Group, Houston, Texas, USA

JAMES A. NORIEGA, DPM, FACFAS, CWSP
Associate Clinical Professor for Family Medicine, Department of Surgery, LSU School of Medicine, Our Lady of Lourdes Hospital, Lafayette, Louisiana, USA

STEPHANIE OEXEMAN, DPM
Fellow, Complex Deformity Correction and Microsurgical Limb Reconstruction, AMITA Health–St. Joseph Hospital, Chicago, Illinois, USA

WILLIAM C. PERRY, DPM
Adjunct Professor of Surgery, University of Cincinnati Medical Center, Attending Podiatrist, Cincinnati VA Medical Center, Veterans Affairs Hospital, Cincinnati, Ohio, USA

DOMINIC A. RIZZO, DPM
Attending Physician and Director of Research, Department of Podiatric Surgery, TriHealth – Bethesda North Hospital, Montgomery, Ohio, USA; Founder and Medical Director, Cincinnati Lower Extremity Reconstructive Institute, Foot and Ankle Specialists of Cincinnati

PEDRO RODRIGUEZ, MD, Plastic and Reconstructive Surgery, OSF Saint Anthony Medical Center, Associate Professor of Surgery, University of Illinois, Rockford, Illinois, USA

ALESSANDRO THIONE, MD, PhD, Consultant Plastic Surgeon, Plastic Surgery and Burn Unit, Department of Plastic Surgery and Burns, Hospital Universitari i Politecnic La Fe, La Fe Hospital, Valencia, Spain

RYAN VAZALES, DPM, Foot and Ankle Surgeon, Department of Orthopedics, Bon Secours-Mercy Health System, Richmond, Virginia, USA

KAITLYN L. WARD, DPM, Fellow, Complex Deformity Correction and Microsurgical Limb Reconstruction, AMITA Health–St. Joseph Hospital, Chicago, Illinois, USA

LOTFY MOHAMED YOUNES, MD, Professor of Orthopedic Surgery and Traumatology, Department of Orthopedic Surgery, Faculty of Medicine, Tanta University, Tanta University Hospital, Tanta, Egypt

Contents

Local and Regional Flaps in Lower Extremity Reconstruction (Muscle and Fasciocutaneous Flaps)

Christopher Bibbo

> The gastrocnemius flap is a versatile flap when muscle, or, muscle and skin is desired for coverage of bone of the proximal one-third of the leg, and about the knee. Both the medial and lateral heads, or both combined, may be used as flaps. Typically, the reach of only the muscle will restrict reach to just below the knee. Release off the medial femoral condyle permits increased reach, and a bit more is obtained by scoring the deep fascia and gently slow expansion of the muscle.

Jose Antonio Delgado Perez, Pedro Rodriguez, Michael D. Liette, and Suhail Masadeh

> Covering soft tissue defects of the tibia is challenging, especially in the presence of underlying osseous trauma. The soleus muscle flap remains the treatment of choice for soft tissue defects in the middle third of the tibia. The flap is reliable and requires a relatively short operative time while maintaining minimal donor site morbidity. However, when the muscle flap is performed without a modified fasciocutaneous composite, it requires a split-thickness skin graft. Muscle flaps have the additional advantage of improving vascularity and fighting infection.

Ahmed Ashraf Fisal, Mohamed Abdel-Hamid Romeih, Lotfy Mohamed Younes, Mahmoud El-Rosasy, Pedro Rodriguez, Michael D. Liette, and Suhail Masadeh

> Wound healing and coverage of soft tissue defects of distal tibia are challenging. Free tissue transfer is treatment of choice for distal tibial defects. However, resources for free tissue transfer are not readily available and they increase morbidity to host. Local and regional flaps play a key role in management of these defects with less demanding or specialized requirements. The soleus muscle flap is the workhorse flap for midtibia soft tissue defects and is used in reverse fashion to reach the distal third of the tibia. Despite minor complications, distally based medial hemisoleus flap is reliable in limb salvage cases.

CLINICS IN PODIATRIC MEDICINE AND SURGERY

SERIES OF RELATED INTEREST

Orthopedic Clinics
Clinics in Sports Medicine
Foot and Ankle Clinics
Physical Medicine and Rehabilitation Clinics

THE CLINICS ARE AVAILABLE ONLINE!
Access your subscription at:
www.theclinics.com

Foreword
Orthoplastics Issue

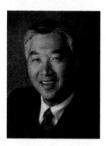

Thomas J. Chang, DPM
Consulting Editor

It is my pleasure to present these next 2 issues on the topic of "Orthoplastics." This is a term capturing the essence of what we already do within our specialty, from the lower leg to the toes. No other specialty focuses equal attention to skin and wounds, to damaged soft tissues, and to correction of bone deformity.

Over the past decade, I have witnessed an explosion of information and courses in lower-extremity plastic surgery, wound care, rotational and advancement skin and muscle flaps, bone surgery, including stabilization and transport and deformity correction. The area of limb salvage has grown exponentially in the amount of knowledge and resources available, and many more compromised limbs are corrected and preserved than ever before.

Several names come to mind when I consider a leader who is passionate on this topic, and clearly Dr Edgardo Rodriguez-Collazo is one of them. When we first met in 1998, I was quickly impressed as he shared his growing experiences with local muscle flaps for difficult wound problems. He is a creative thinker and talented surgeon who early on devoted his career to the area of Orthoplastics. I applaud his vision and his contributions to our profession and to lower-extremity surgeons globally.

I believe this collection of topics will be an authoritative resource in the area of lower-extremity Orthoplastics for the future. It is my hope these next 2 issues will serve as a mini textbook and invaluable reference for anyone interested in taking limb salvage to a higher level. Drs Rodriguez-Collazo and Masadeh have brought together a stellar internationally diverse group of educators in the world of Orthoplastics. These approaches again validate the value of a multidisciplinary approach in how we can achieve greater success with this difficult subset of problems and patients.

Clin Podiatr Med Surg 37 (2020) xiii–xiv
https://doi.org/10.1016/j.cpm.2020.07.011
0891-8422/20/© 2020 Published by Elsevier Inc.

I trust this will be a worthwhile addition to your library.

Thomas J. Chang, DPM
Redwood Orthopedic Surgery Associates
208 Concourse Boulevard
Santa Rosa, CA 95403, USA

E-mail address:
thomaschang14@comcast.net

Preface

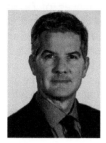
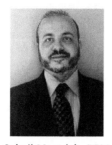

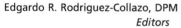

Edgardo R. Rodriguez-Collazo, DPM   Suhail Masadeh, DPM

Editors

The inception of the American Microsurgical and Orthoplastic Society led to the assembly of the most talented national and international physicians with a passion for lower-limb reconstruction. The primary goal of the group was to provide unrestricted education across multiple specialties to address the frequent and challenging complications in this area of reconstructive surgery. During World War II, surgeons from general, orthopedic and plastics combined their expertise to manage the devastating effects seen in the upper extremity. This ultimately led to the emergence of an upper extremity and hand surgical specialty. The ability to manage complex small and large bone fractures as well as soft tissue defects with tendon, nerve, and vessel injuries improved outcomes for functional limb restoration. Our hope was to inspire the development and advancement of a lower-limb specialist.

The role of Podiatric surgery is often the key to achieving limb salvage. The advances in our profession with subspecialized training in orthoplastic techniques have produced skillful surgeons capable of handling complex limb reconstruction. Our collaborative work with other surgical specialties has drastically improved patient outcomes and underscores the valuable role of the podiatric surgeon as an integral part of the medical team.

The advancement of technology has created an open educational platform and collaborative work across borders and the globe. The inspiration for this issue of *Clinics in Podiatric Medicine and Surgery* was an open educational philosophy and the belief in high-quality education and resources for everyone in the world. This was evident by the collaborative work of the podiatric, orthopedic, plastic, and microvascular surgeons who contributed to the articles of this issue. In this issue of *Clinics in Podiatric Medicine and Surgery*, a broad overview is provided for the various techniques available for soft tissue and osseous reconstruction of the lower limb. We divided the articles in a concise way to cover local and regional muscle and fasciocutaneous flaps from the proximal leg to the forefoot to provide solutions for these difficult problems. We provided several cadaveric and clinical examples to illustrate the technical components of the various procedures included within this issue. In addition, a brief overview is provided of orthobiologics and their role in the reconstructive ladder,

Clin Podiatr Med Surg 37 (2020) xv–xvi
https://doi.org/10.1016/j.cpm.2020.07.008
0891-8422/20/© 2020 Published by Elsevier Inc.

podiatric.theclinics.com

the role of reconstructive amputations of the lower limb, with an emphasis on preservation of function and length and the treatment options for segmental bone defects.

I would like to thank all the contributing authors of this special issue of the *Clinics in Podiatric Medicine and Surgery* highlighting the major influences of Dr Edgardo Rodriguez-Collazo, Dr Pedro Rodriguez, and Dr Christopher Bibbo. These amazing physicians are always at the forefront of education and have inspired old and new practitioners alike. I would also like to extend a special thanks to our international faculty from Egypt, Spain, and Mexico for their constant collaboration and contribution to the high quality and equality of education across the globe. Last, I would like to recognize and thank the countless individuals who donated their bodies for their selfless act and their impact on education and scientific advancements.

Edgardo R. Rodriguez-Collazo, DPM
AMITA Saint Joseph Hospital
Attn: Podiatric Fellowship Office
2913 N Commonwealth Avenue
Chicago, IL 60657, USA

Suhail Masadeh, DPM
231 Albert Sabin Way, ML 0513
Cincinnati, OH 45276, USA

E-mail addresses:
egodpm@gmail.com (E.R. Rodriguez-Collazo)
smasadehdpm@gmail.com (S. Masadeh)

Local and Regional Flaps in Lower Extremity Reconstruction (Muscle and Fasciocutaneous Flaps)

The Gastrocnemius Flap for Lower Extremity Reconstruction

Christopher Bibbo, DO, DPM

KEYWORDS

- Gastrocnemius flap • Medial muscle flap

KEY POINTS

- The medial or lateral heads, or both combined, may be used as flaps.
- The indication for a skin island with the gastrocnemius flap is when an extra-durable layer of tissue is desired over a defect, such as when there is an exposed total knee prosthesis, or for proximal tibial plateau fracture implants that are critical and cannot be removed.
- Large areas of soft tissue loss of the leg greater length may be managed by a combined medial gastrocnemius and soleus rotation flap construct.

The gastrocnemius flap is a versatile flap when muscle or muscle and skin are desired for coverage of bone of the proximal one-third of the leg and about the knee. Both the medial and lateral heads, or both combined, may be used as flaps. The medial gastrocnemius has a greater excursion, mass, and perforator distribution.[1–4] Typically, the reach of only the muscle restricts reach to just below the knee. Release off the medial femoral condyle permits increased reach, and a bit more is obtained by scoring the deep fascia and gently slowing expansion of the muscle. When a skin island is added (myocutaneous medial gastrocnemius flap), however, the reach can be extended both proximally over the knee and distally over the anterior leg. The lateral head is not as reliable to support a skin island.

OPERATIVE TECHNIQUE
Medial Gastrocnemius Muscle Flap

A medial, midline posterior, or respective medial midaxial incision may be utilized (**Fig. 1**). With the midline posterior approach, dissection is carried to the deep fascia; the short saphenous vein and sural nerve are preserved. With both the medial and lateral midaxial approaches, dissection is carried to the edge of the muscle and aponeurosis and a plane developed just above the muscle; a large retractor

Foot and Ankle Surgery, Plastic Reconstructive and Microsurgery, Orthopaedic Trauma, and MSK Infection Services, Rubin Institute for Advanced Orthopedics, Sinai Hospital of Baltimore, 2401 West Belvedere Avenue, Baltimore, MD 21215, USA
E-mail address: cbibbo@lifebridgehealth.org

Clin Podiatr Med Surg 37 (2020) 609–619
https://doi.org/10.1016/j.cpm.2020.07.002
0891-8422/20/© 2020 Elsevier Inc. All rights reserved.

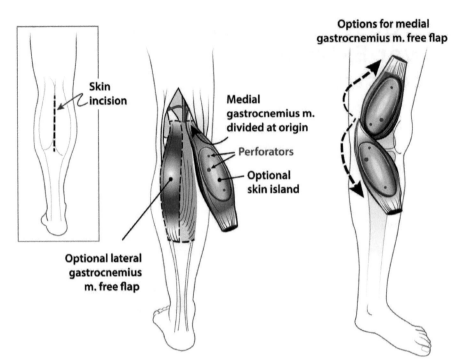

Fig. 1. Illustration of midline incision, division of median raphe and hemisection of the Achilles tendon. Skin island over the medial head is nourished by sural perforating vessels. The flap may be rotated as needed with the skin island. (With Permission. Copyright 2020, Rubin Institute for Advanced Orthopedics, Sinai Hospital of Baltimore.)

is needed to retract the posterior tissues. The median raphe is identified and the muscle head(s) isolated. The median raphe is split, and the split carried medial or lateral, depending on muscle head being used (**Fig. 2**A). A submuscular plane is created easily by finger sweeping, revealing the underlying soleus muscle (**Fig. 2**B). Medially, the relatively constant sural cutaneous perforators need division; the lateral sural perforators are small and usually taken with standard monopolar or bipolar dissection.

Insetting of the flap may be performed by undermining the skin and subcutaneous tissues, creating a tunnel 2-times to 2.5-times the width of the flap (to accommodate flap swelling), and the flap is transferred though the tunnel (**Fig. 3**). When sufficient room cannot be made, there should be no hesitation to perform a back-cut and lay the muscle flap in the back-cut, secured into the recipient bed; then, the local tissue is gently sutured to the edge of the flap (**Fig. 4**). The author prefers insetting by placing a suture in the distal aponeurosis tail of the flap and drawing the tail into the subcutaneous space of the recipient bed, with a suture knot exteriorized approximately 2 cm away from the flap/recipient bed suture line; a flat drain may be placed under the flap prior to full inset. When additional reach is needed, the deep fascia of the muscle may be scored transversely (**Fig. 5**). Likewise, the fascia also may be scored transversely and longitudinally, allowing expansion of flap in length and width (Bibbo technique). Both these 2 techniques are gentle maneuvers—the muscle may tear in half if performed too aggressively. Any further length may be obtained by progressive release of the attachment fascia of gastrocnemius origin—this is the only time the vascular pedicle is visualized, ensuring the vessels are not strangulated by

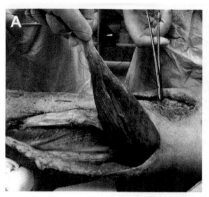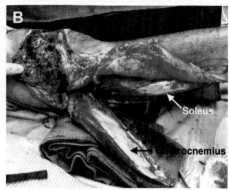

Fig. 2. (*A*) Simple exposure and isolation of the medial head of the gastrocnemius muscle. (*B*) A wide-open exposure of the harvest of the medial gastrocnemius flap, required for proximal release. Note the underlying soleus. (With Permission. Copyright 2020, Main Street Enterprises, LLC, DBA Global Medicus.)

overzealous stretching of the vessels. Upon visualization of the pedicle, the decision to neurotinize the muscle by dividing the sural motor nerve is made, because patients may experience fasciculation or spasm of the muscle with knee flexion. The author has observed this in fewer than one-third of patients; the response is mild and abates by 6 months to 12 months and does not routinely divide the nerve, unless extended muscle release is prevented by intraoperative contraction of the muscle.

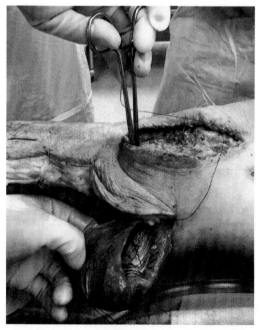

Fig. 3. Creation of a wide tunnel and transfer of the muscle flap through the tunnel. (With Permission. Copyright 2020, Main Street Enterprises, LLC, DBA Global Medicus.)

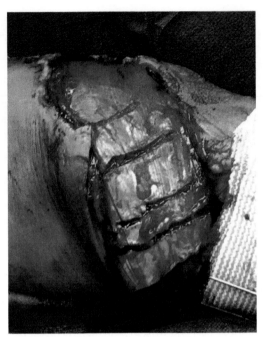

Fig. 4. Medial gastrocnemius passed along a back-cut leading to the donor defect—this technique may be thought of as laying the flap into an extended defect area. (With Permission. Copyright 2020, Main Street Enterprises, LLC, DBA Global Medicus.)

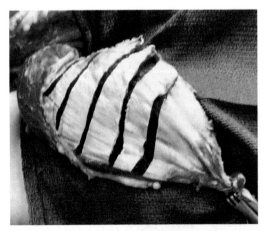

Fig. 5. Scoring of the gastrocnemius fascia on the under surface of the muscle to increase flap length. The scoring should be only through the fascia—excessive penetration into the muscle disrupts the flap. (With Permission. Copyright 2020, Main Street Enterprises, LLC, DBA Global Medicus.)

The muscle is either skin-grafted immediately (**Fig. 6**) or grafted in a delayed fashion using negative-pressure wound dressings and a neodermal matrix. Delaying skin grafts often are used to improve cosmetic appearance (contour and depth match) and promote a more durable layer of superficial tissues over the muscle. The donor site is closed to decrease the potential space in multiple layers, with drains placed in at least 1 level. The site of the aponeurotic partial hemisection is repaired with a robust check-rein stitch (the author uses braided absorbable suture only for tendon surgery). Donor site closure is meticulous, performed in multiple layers over closed suction drains.

Medial Gastrocnemius Myocutaneous Flap

The indications for a skin island with the gastrocnemius flap (see **Fig. 1**) are when an extra-durable layer of tissue is desired over a defect, such as when there is an exposed total knee prosthesis, or for proximal tibial plateau fracture implants that are critical and cannot be removed (**Fig. 7**). Additionally, the addition of a skin island may extend flap reach when defect location exceeds that of the muscle. The medial head of the gastrocnemius reliably carries a skin island when the skin perforator(s) have an audible Doppler signal. The sural perforator vessel emanates from the medial sural artery, follows an intramuscular course, and continues through the fascial planes to supply the overlying skin (see **Fig. 7**). This vessel is searched for by Doppler beginning in the upper one-third of the muscle, working proximal to distal sweeping side to side. There usually is at least 1 dominant vessel; smaller vessels may be present.[1-4] The size of the skin island is designed to fit the length, width, and orientation of the wound; skin islands may be vertical, oblique, or horizontal (**Figs. 8**A and **9**). Empirically, the author usually designs the island no greater than 75% of the length and width of the medial gastrocnemius head. When vertical skin island length desired, the author takes a few centimeters below the most distant extend of the muscle belly,

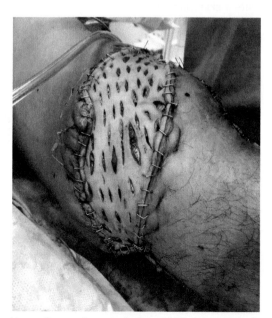

Fig. 6. Immediate skin graft over the muscle flap. (With Permission. Copyright 2020, Main Street Enterprises, LLC, DBA Global Medicus.)

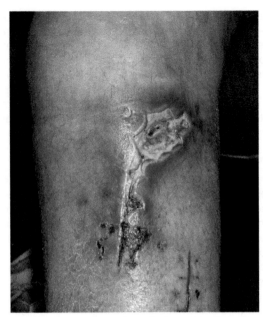

Fig. 7. Proximal plateau wound that extends to the knee joint line. Use of a skin island may assist with reach and provide a more durable flap composed of all-natural tissue composites. (With Permission. Copyright 2020, Main Street Enterprises, LLC, DBA Global Medicus.)

occasionally extending over the triceps surae aponeurosis—the author recommends an exhaustive progressive Doppler examination as such a distal dissection proceeds. The key point to elevate a skin island is that the skin island tracing must be followed carefully so as to not exclude the perforator, and the dissection must not undermine the soft tissue attachment to the gastrocnemius muscle (**Fig. 8**B). Flap insetting

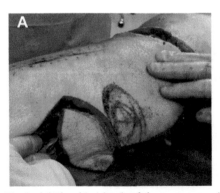
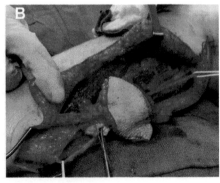

Fig. 8. (*A*) The skin islands of the gastrocnemius myocutaneous flap may be vertical, oblique, or, as shown, horizontal. The design and orientation must be planned carefully to not only accommodate the defect shape but also take into consideration the final position as dictated by the path of inset. (*B*) Photo illustrating that the skin island must remain attached to the underlying muscle. Note the course of the sural nerve (held by the vessel loop), which is variable in depth relation to the muscle flap. (With Permission. Copyright 2020, Main Street Enterprises, LLC, DBA Global Medicus.)

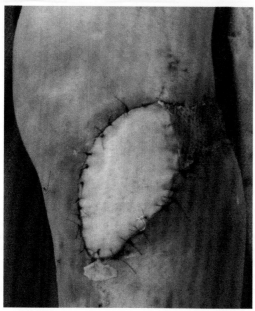

Fig. 9. Final inset of a medial gastrocnemius myocutaneous flap, designed as to fit an obli-que orientation. (With Permission. Copyright 2020, Main Street Enterprises, LLC, DBA Global Medicus.)

may be performed through a tunnel or via a back-cut (with a skin graft overlaying the exposed muscle that does not fill the target defect). The reach of the flap now may extend to the level of the proximal plateau (see **Fig. 9**), the patella, and the mid/distal anterior leg. Based on the geometry and orientation of the skin island, the flap donor site is closed primarily via standard technique via relaxing incisions or, in difficult donor sites (primarily in obese patients), neodermal matrix/negative-pressure dressing/skin graft or skin-grafted (**Fig. 10**).

Lateral Gastrocnemius Flap

After either a midline or lateral-midline approach, sharp dissection is carried to the fas-cia. The incision is carried proximally to the neck of the fibula and the common pero-neal nerve released. The nerve should not be manipulated with maneuvers, such as an encircling Penrose drain clamped with a hemostat; if a point of identification is desired, a Penrose or vessel loop may be paced around the nerve without a clamp. Identical to the medial head, the aponeurosis is split and carried out to the lateral edge of the mus-cle, leaving a tail of fascia with the lateral head. The muscle is rotated over the com-mon peroneal nerve and inset.

Combined Medial and Lateral Gastrocnemius Flap

When there exists significant loss of the soft tissue envelope of the proximal one-third of the leg, or a combined medial-lateral, with or without anterior wound, the medial and lateral gastrocnemius muscle may be employed simultaneously. A combined medial-lateral gastrocnemius flap configuration also may include a medial flap skin island to ensure coverage needs of the distal extent of the flap (**Fig. 11**). The plantar flexion function of the triceps surae is diminished slightly, but the long toe flexors and the

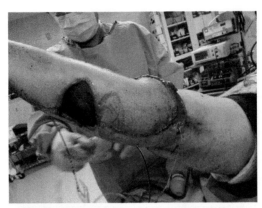

Fig. 10. Large donor site defect after a medial gastrocnemius myocutaneous flap. Flaps may require a combination of insetting techniques. Note that this flap has been both tunneled under the donor site suture line as well as inset into a back-cut. The underlying soleus muscle and exposed gastrocnemius may be skin-grafted or, as in this instance, covered with a neodermal ingrowth matrix with/without a negative-pressure dressing, followed by a delayed skin graft. This technique improved the cosmetic appearance of the flap surface, and the door site. Note that the extensive dissection merits 3 drains. (With Permission. Copyright 2020, Main Street Enterprises, LLC, DBA Global Medicus.)

posterior tibial tendon contribute to flexion strength—the author has not found it necessary to employ an immediate or delayed tendon transfer.

Combined Medial Gastrocnemius and Soleus Flaps

Large areas of soft tissue loss of the leg greater length may be managed by a combined medial gastrocnemius and soleus rotation flap construct (**Fig. 12**). This technique is facilitated best by a medial midline incision and a counter-posterior midline incision. A medial hemisoleus or full soleus flap is elevated; weakness becomes more apparent with use of the entire soleus, long-term management of which with an ankle-foot orthosis usually is necessary.

External Fixation and Gastrocnemius Flaps

External fixation with flaps (flap and frame concept) was first utilized by Bibbo in 2006.[5,6] Virtually all extremity flaps may find utilization of external fixation beneficial for off-loading, joint stabilization, or concomitant deformity correction. With the gastrocnemius flap(s), if severe weakness is anticipated after a combined medial-lateral flap combination due to the presence of weakened deep posterior compartment muscles, the application of a 5o equinus external fixator may mitigate the development of weakened plantar-flexion strength (relative calcaneal gait). When the gastrocnemius flap crossed the knee or knee motion may compromise flap healing, a transarticular external fixator can assist with flap stabilization while still allowing weight bearing (**Fig. 13**). A complete description of external fixation with flap surgery is provided in A Novel Technique of External Fixation for Immediate Post-Operative Ambulation and Protection of Soft Tissue Reconstructions ("Bibbo Flap & Frame" Technique) in Volume 2.

Drains are maintained until the output is less than 20 mL per drain, for 2 consecutive 8-hour periods. The incision line must be without tension for 6 weeks to 8 weeks. In some instances, this may require knee immobilization. In most cases, however, full

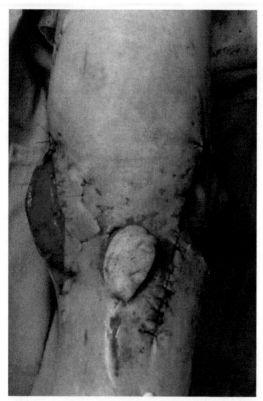

Fig. 11. Soft tissue coverage of dehisced medial, lateral, and anterior knee incisions after open reduction and internal fixation of a bicondylar tibial plateau fracture. A combination of a medial myocutanous and muscle-only lateral gastrocnemius flaps was employed. The skin island of the medial flap was used to cover a critical defect overlying the patellar tendon and its' insertion onto the tibial tubercle. (With Permission. Copyright 2020, Main Street Enterprises, LLC, DBA Global Medicus.)

weight bearing is permitted. After an initial 2 weeks, compressive dressings are instituted. Skin grafts are cared for by surgeon preference. The author routinely leaves sutures in place 4 weeks. Showering is permitted after skin grafts have matured. Nutritional support is continued throughout the perioperative period. Formal physical therapy begins in the hospital with balanced quadriceps-hamstring isometric strengthening as well as ankle isometrics. Complex musculoskeletal conditions existing along with the flap are cared for as required and prioritization of care is determined by the surgeon. After the flap has healed, routine surveillance is at 6 months, then at 12 months, and then as needed.

Complications

Complications are not frequent but include hematoma (#1), suture line dehiscence, infection, and flap loss. Each is managed in standard fashions. It cannot be stresses enough that multiple layer closure over drains(s) (see **Fig. 10; Fig. 14**) is critical, because patients normally are placed on anticoagulants postoperatively and may continue to bleed into the leg. Revision of the flap may include advancement and rein-set, débridement, and possibly a new revision flap. Infections are managed by culture-

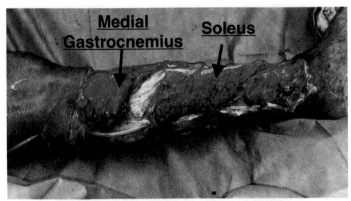

Fig. 12. The combination of a medial gastrocnemius flap with a soleus flap used to cover the tibia for a wound extending from the proximal leg to ankle. This may result in noticeable plantarflexion weakness; thus, an external fixator 5° of plantar flexion may be used, which also protects skin grafting (one of the Bibbo flap and frame concepts). Limb rehabilitation included the use of a postoperative ankle foot arthrosis. (With Permission. Copyright 2020, Main Street Enterprises, LLC, DBA Global Medicus.)

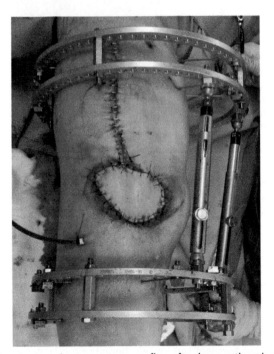

Fig. 13. A medial gastrocnemius myocutaneous flap after knee arthroplasty explant with a soft tissue defect over the anterior proximal tibia, patellar tendon and tibial tubercle. The flap and explanted knee are stabilized by a locked transarticular external fixator (in the process of assembly), which also allows weight-bearing mobilization (Bibbo flap and frame concept). Again, note the use of a drain. (With Permission. Copyright 2020, Main Street Enterprises, LLC, DBA Global Medicus.)

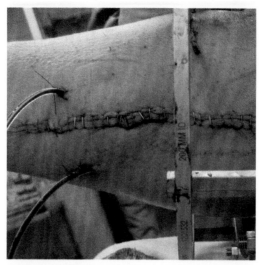

Fig. 14. Drains are essential in flap surgery. A hematoma under a flap may result in infection, suture line dehiscence, or pedicle compression, all of which may impart a flap failure. The drain technique in this photo illustrates drains at different wound depths (deep and superficial), a distal exit for gravity pooling of blood while the patient is in the upright position during mobilization. The author secures all drains with sutures. (With Permission. Copyright 2020, Main Street Enterprises, LLC, DBA Global Medicus.)

specific antibiotics; the author continues antibiotics with flap necrosis until all devitalized tissue is healthy. Osteomyelitis is managed for 8 weeks of antibiotics with repeat operative cultures determining the course of any additional antibiotic treatment. When flap loss is incomplete, successful salvage may be met by tangential débridement and negative-pressure dressing, followed by skin grafting. The need for secondary flaps is uncommon, but when complete flap failure occurs, free tissue transfers become an indication.

DISCLOSURE

The author has nothing to disclose.

REFERENCES

1. Hupkens P, Westland PB, Schijns W, et al. Medial lower leg perforators: an anatomical study of their distribution andcharacteristics. Microsurgery 2017;37(4):319–26.
2. Thione A, Valdatta L, Buoro M, et al. The medial sural artery perforators: anatomic basis for a surgical plan. Ann Plast Surg 2004;53(3):250–5.
3. Hallock GG. Anatomic basis of the gastrocnemius perforator-based flap. Ann Plast Surg 2001;47(5):517–22.
4. Wong MZ, Wong CH, Tan BK, et al. Surgical anatomy of the medial sural artery perforator flap. J Reconstr Microsurg 2012;28(8):555–60.
5. Bibbo C. A novel technique of external fixation for immediate post-operative ambulation and protection of soft tissue reconstructions ("Flap & Frame" technique). Clin Pod Med Surg, in press.
6. Bibbo C. Foot and ankle surgery for chronic non-healing wounds. Surg Clin North Am, in press.

Medial Hemisoleus Flap for Middle Third of the Tibia Defects

Jose Antonio Delgado Perez, MD[a,1], Pedro Rodriguez, MD[b], Michael D. Liette, DPM[c], Suhail Masadeh, DPM[d],*

KEYWORDS

- Soleus flap • Lower limb reconstruction • Tibial wound • Muscle flap

KEY POINTS

- Open wounds of the tibia are associated with a high rate of complications and morbidity.
- High-energy injuries to the tibia are often associated with severe soft tissue damage.
- The soleus muscle flap is the flap of choice for soft tissue reconstruction of the middle third of the tibia.
- The soleus flap provides reliable coverage with a short operative time and minimal donor site morbidity.
- Muscle flaps improve vascularity to the wound sites reconstructed and aid in the treatment of osteomyelitis.

INTRODUCTION

Open wounds of the tibia may be caused by trauma, surgery, or chronic ulceration. These wounds often lead to significant morbidity and have the potential for limb loss. The anteromedial portion of the tibia lacks significant soft tissue coverage and is susceptible to open wounds that may lead to bone exposure and subsequent infection. Open fractures can occur as a result of high-energy trauma or from low-energy injuries, in the case of osteoporotic fractures. Soft tissue injuries associated with tibial fractures are an independent factor for developing delayed unions and nonunions, with a range from 9% to 12%.[1] The high prevalence and severe morbidity

[a] National Institute of Pediatrics, Mexico City, Mexico; [b] Plastic and Reconstructive Surgery, OSF Saint Anthony Medical Center, 698 Featherstone Road, Rockford, IL 61107, USA; [c] University of Cincinnati Medical Center, 231 Albert Sabin Way, ML 0513, Cincinnati, OH 45276, USA; [d] University of Cincinnati Medical Center, Cincinnati Veteran Affairs Medical Center, 231 Albert Sabin Way, ML 0513, Cincinnati, OH 45276, USA
[1] Present address: PO Box 04530, 3700-cinsurgents sur av. Insurgentes cuicuiclo, Mexico City, Mexico.
* Corresponding author.
E-mail address: masadesb@uc.edu

Clin Podiatr Med Surg 37 (2020) 621–630
https://doi.org/10.1016/j.cpm.2020.05.001
0891-8422/20/Published by Elsevier Inc.

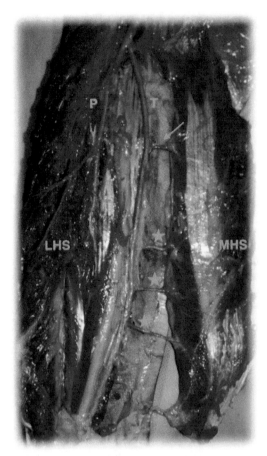

Fig. 1. Lateral hemiseoleus (LHS), the medial hemisoleus (MHS), and their respective vascular supplies arising from either the peroneal artery (P) or the posterior tibial artery (T). The posterior tibial artery supplies the medial aspect of the muscle through one major pedicle (*arrow*) and several minor pedicles (*stars*). (*Courtesy of* S. Masadeh, DPM, Cincinnati, OH.)

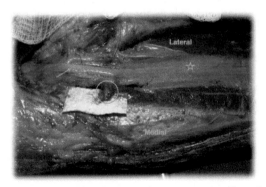

Fig. 2. The tibial nerve (*arrow*), the fascia and accompanying fat of the neurovascular bundle (*star*), and the dominant perforator of the posterior tibial artery with its accompanying venae comitantes (*circle*). (*Courtesy of* S. Masadeh, DPM, Cincinnati, OH.)

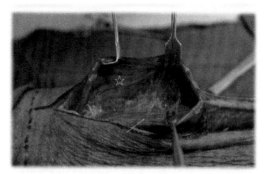

Fig. 3. Separation of the soleus muscle (*arrow*) from the overlying gastrocnemius muscle (*star*) by retracting the gastrocnemius superior and lateral. (*Courtesy of* S. Masadeh, DPM, Cincinnati, OH.)

associated with open wounds of the tibia dictate the need for early wound coverage to minimize complications. Local muscle flaps improve wound vascularity, provide bulk, and limit bacterial colonization and infection.[2–5] They additionally promote rapid collagen deposition and early tissue regeneration.[2–4] The soleus muscle flap has proved to be an excellent treatment option for soft tissue coverage in the middle third of the tibia.[6]

ANATOMY

The soleus muscle is a bipennate muscle that originates within the superficial posterior compartment of the lower extremity, deep or anterior to the gastrocnemius muscle.[7,8] It is divided into medial and lateral heads that originate from the posterior surface of the tibia and fibula, respectively. It functions to plantarflex the ankle along with the gastrocnemius muscle as they join to form the achilles tendon. The 2 heads are conjoined proximally and separated distally by an intramuscular septum, otherwise known as the central raphe.[7,8] The hemisoleus is classified as a type II muscle according to the Mathes and Nahai classification.[9] Vascular supply is composed of one dominant pedicle accompanied by several minor pedicles supplying the vasculature to the muscle (**Fig. 1**).[9] The blood supply to the medial half of the muscle arises from perforators originating from the posterior tibial artery. The lateral half is supplied by

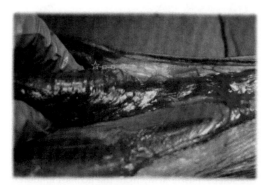

Fig. 4. Visualized is the isolation and separation of the conjoined tendon (*star*). (*Courtesy of* S. Masadeh, DPM, Cincinnati, OH.)

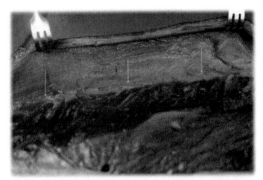

Fig. 5. The soleus remains attached to the tibia (*arrows*) during flap dissection and allows for traction/countertraction maneuvers to assist in elevation. (*Courtesy of* S. Masadeh, DPM, Cincinnati, OH.)

perforators from the peroneal artery with both halves innervated by the motor branch of the tibial nerve (**Fig. 2**).[7,8]

SURGICAL TECHNIQUE
Medial Approach

The patient is placed in the supine position with a bump under the contralateral side to allow for external rotation of the extremity. The medial boarder of the tibia is identified and the cleavage point between the gastrocnemius and soleus is located, which is distinct and palpable even in obese patients. This cleavage point, which is typically 2 to 3 cm from the tibial tuberosity, is outlined from the proximal tibia to the level of the medial malleolus and will serve as the anatomic location for incision placement. Care must be taken to identify and preserve the great saphenous vein and nerve during dissection, as preservation of this vein aids in superficial venous outflow, important in postoperative edema control. Alternatively, if a soft tissue defect is present close to the planned incision line, the defect is extended proximally and distally in the same fashion to incorporate the defect within the surgical plan. The incision is then made through the skin and subcutaneous fascia to the level of the deep fascia. Bridging

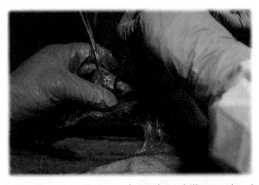

Fig. 6. Reflection of the soleus muscle away from the achilles tendon (*star*), preserving the achilles tendon in the process to maintain plantarflexion strength. (*Courtesy of* S. Masadeh, DPM, Cincinnati, OH.)

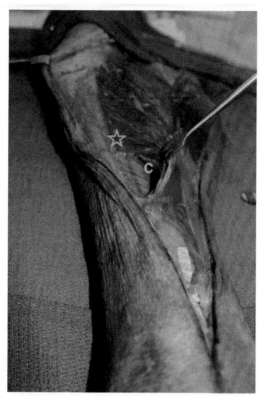

Fig. 7. The "C-point" (C). As the soleus curves from its fibrous attachment to the tibia (*star*), it provides a distinct dissection plane, which allows for atraumatic separation of the soleus from the flexor digitorum longus muscle while preserving the thin fascia overlying the tibial neurovascular bundle. (*Courtesy of* S. Masadeh, DPM, Cincinnati, OH.)

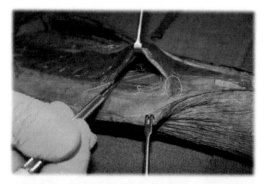

Fig. 8. The "C-point." As the soleus curves from its fibrous attachment to the tibia, it provides a distinct dissection plane, which allows for atraumatic separation of the soleus from the flexor digitorum longus muscle while preserving the thin fascia overlying the tibial neurovascular bundle. Arrow is pointing to the fibrous attachment of the C-point on the tibia and the circle points to the thin fascia over the neurovascular bundle. (*Courtesy of* S. Masadeh, DPM, Cincinnati, OH.)

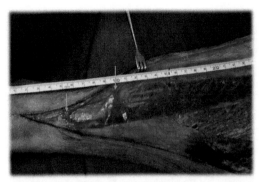

Fig. 9. The distal perforators supply the medial hemisoleus. During dissection, it is critical to preserve as many of the perforating branches but continue to allow for an adequate arc of rotation of the muscle to cover the soft tissue deficit without tension. The solid arrows point to the distal perforators of the medial hemisoleus and the dotted line points toward the proximal perforator. (*Courtesy of* S. Masadeh, DPM, Cincinnati, OH.)

veins are ligated and the deep fascia is identified in the proximal two-thirds of the leg as it becomes more superficial distally. The deep fascia is then incised to identify and isolate the gastrocnemius muscle, and the fasciotomy is carried distally to the level of the medial malleolus. The minor perforators are more superficial within the distal third of the leg and care must be taken to avoid injury to these during dissection.

The gastrocnemius muscle is then gently reflected superior and lateral and separated from the soleus muscle (**Fig. 3**). Although the dissection plane between the gastrocnemius and soleus is considered "avascular," care must be taken to identify and ligate the direct muscular arterial branches. The gastrocnemius is further elevated past the central raphe of the soleus, and the dissection is carried from proximal to distal until the conjoined tendon of the achilles is reached (**Fig. 4**). Once the gastrocnemius is isolated and fully separated, attention is again directed to the soleus. The soleus attachment to the tibia is maintained during flap elevation, to allow for traction and countertraction to facilitate dissection as the distal soleus is detached from the achilles tendon (**Fig. 5**). Care must be taken during this maneuver to preserve the aponeurosis of the tendon, which is often very thin.

Once isolated from the achilles tendon, the distal part of the soleus, with its aponeurosis intact, is cut so as to avoid injury to the achilles tendon **Fig. 6**. As the soleus

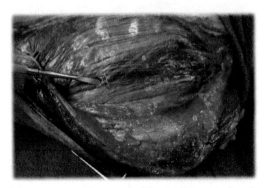

Fig. 10. Elevation of the gastrocnemius muscle (G) past the central raphe of the soleus (S) to expose the central raphe (*star*) and the intermuscular artery within. (*Courtesy of* S. Masadeh, DPM, Cincinnati, OH.)

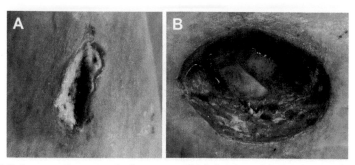

Fig. 11. (*A*) Preoperative wound after open tibial fracture. (*B*) Postdebridement of the wound to healthy bleeding margins with notable exposed tibia within the wound bed. (*Courtesy of* S. Masadeh, DPM, Cincinnati, OH.)

curves from its fibrous attachment to the tibia, it provides a distinct dissection plane that is termed the "C-point," which allows for atraumatic separation of the soleus muscle from the fascia of the deep posterior compartment (**Figs. 7** and **8**). The major and minor pedicles providing the vasculature to the soleus are then identified. It is paramount to preserve as many of these perforators as possible while allowing enough rotation to reach the defect to improve the survivability of the flap (**Fig. 9**).[10] The soleus muscle is then split longitudinally just lateral to the central raphe, preserving the intermuscular artery, which may aid in flap perfusion through communicating vessels from the contralateral peroneal artery, as visualized in **Fig. 10**. The muscle is then rotated and inset into the defect without tension. To obtain additional expansion of the muscle, the soleus fascia may be scored or removed, which can increase the reach of the flap so as to maintain a tension-free inset. A split-thickness skin graft is harvested and secured to the flap for muscle coverage. Alternatively, if the flap is questionable, temporization with a dermal regenerative template and negative pressure wound

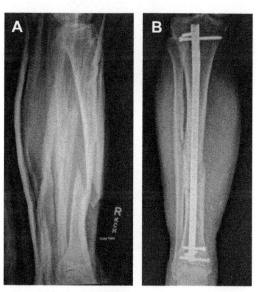

Fig. 12. (*A*) Preoperative midshaft tibial fracture and the (*B*) postoperative fracture stabilization using an intramedullary rod for fixation. (*Courtesy of* S. Masadeh, DPM, Cincinnati, OH.)

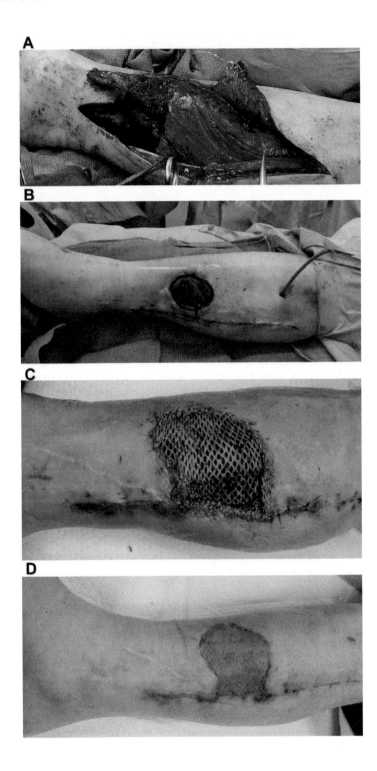

therapy may aid in successful skin grafting at a later date. A drain is placed between the superficial and deep posterior compartments at the harvest site to allow for fluid management. It should be noted that before flap elevation, surgical sites should be thoroughly debrided and any necessary fracture stabilization performed (**Figs. 11–13**).

ANALYSIS/DISCUSSION

Soft tissue injuries with bone exposure involving the middle third of the tibia can pose a significant clinical challenge. Wounds associated with open tibial fractures often have significant morbidity associated with them, as they have demonstrated infection rates approaching 40% and nonunion rates as high as 23%.[11] The soleus muscle flap, as first described by *Tobin* in 1985, has often been used for the treatment of these wounds.[12] The 2 heads of the muscle have independent blood supply, allowing for the great versatility of this flap. Utilization of the entire muscle is not necessary and limits the arc of rotation; therefore, the preferred method is to split the muscle past the central raphe to improve the reach of the flap by up to 15 cm.[12,13] Harvesting half of the muscle, and preserving the lateral hemisoleus, retains plantarflexion strength, although this is reduced compared with preoperative levels.[10,13,14] The medial hemisoleus has consistent blood supply including dominant and minor pedicles with improved arc of rotation and is technically less demanding to harvest than the lateral hemisoleus.[15] Similar to other wounds and flap assessment, careful evaluation of the patient and vascular perfusion is critical.

Soft tissue debridement and fracture stabilization via internal or external fixation are additional key components for successful soft tissue stabilization after flap harvest. In cases of high-energy trauma, the muscle may not be a viable option for reconstruction if it is within the zone of injury and the muscular perforators or the muscle itself is damaged.[15] Therefore, a thorough vascular workup whether via duplex doppler, computed tomography angiography, magnetic resonance angiography, or angiography may be warranted.[16] A study performed by Thornton and colleagues analyzed the cost and survivability of free flaps as compared with the medial hemisoleus flap for the management of distal tibial wounds. They found a decrease in the length of stay in the hospital, operative time, and costs when using the medial hemisoleus as well as equivalent postoperative outcomes in cosmetic and fracture healing between the 2 groups[17]; this further supports the use of local rotational muscle flaps in the management of these defects. Many variations of this flap have been described, including the use of an osteomuscular flap and basing the flap distally.[15] Furthermore, the medial hemisoleus can be used with the gastrocnemius flap when a larger defect is present.

CLINICAL CARE POINTS

- The soleus muscle flap provides a reliable option for coverage of complex middle third of the tibia defects.
- The 2 heads of the muscle have independent and consistent blood supply.

Fig. 13. (*A*) The elevation and rotation of the medial hemisoleus flap to cover exposed tibial fracture after fracture stabilization was obtained. (*B*) Flap is then inset tension-free, and a drain is placed in the posterior compartment to avoid hematoma formation. (*C*) A split-thickness skin graft is used to provide coverage of the now rotated hemisoleus flap. (*D*) Healed medial hemisoleus flap after successful incorporation of split-thickness skin graft. (*Courtesy of* S. Masadeh, DPM, Cincinnati, OH.)

- The medial hemisoleus has a good arch of rotation, with intermediate technical demands that do not require microvascular anastomosis.
- There is little donor site morbidity with preservation of ankle plantar flexion.
- The flap requires a skin graft to achieve complete soft tissue coverage with acceptable cosmetic outcome.

DISCLOSURE

The authors have nothing to disclose.

REFERENCES

1. Schmidt AH, Finkemeier CG, Tornetta P. Treatment of closed tibial fractures. J Bone Joint Surg 2003;85-A(2):352–68.
2. Calderon W, Chang N, MAthes SJ. Comparison of the effect of bacterial inoculation in musculocutaneous and fasciocutaneous flaps. Plast Reconstr Surg 1986; 77(5):785–94.
3. Chang N, Mathes SJ. Comparison of the effect of bacterial inoculation in musculocutaneous and random-pattern flaps. Plast Reconstr Surg 1982;70(1):1–10.
4. Gosain A, Chang N, Mathes S, et al. A Study of the relationship between blood flow and bacterial inoculation in musculocutaneous and fasciocutaneous flaps. Plast Reconstr Surg 1990;86(6):1163.
5. Klebuc M, Menn Z. Muscle flaps and their role in limb salvage. Methodist Debakey Cardiovasc J 2013;9:95–9.
6. Ahmad I, Khurram M. Hemisoleus muscle flap in the reconstruction of exposed bones in the lower limb. J Wound Care 2013;22(11):635–42.
7. Kelikian AS, Sarrafian SK. Sarrafians anatomy of the foot and ankle, 3rd edition. Philadelphia: Lippincott Williams & Wilkins. p. 326–36.
8. Raveendran SS, Kumaragama KGJL. Arterial supply of the soleus muscle: anatomical study of fifty lower limbs. Clin Anat 2003;16:248–52.
9. Mathes SJ, Nahai F. Classification of the vascular anatomy of muscle: experimental and clinical correlation. Plast Reconstr Surg 1981;67:177–87.
10. Pu LIQ. Successful soft-tissue coverage of a tibial wound in the distal third of the leg with a medial hemisoleus muscle flap. Plast Reconstr Surg 2005;115(1): 245–51.
11. Kohlprath R, Assal M, Uckay I, et al. Open fracture of the tibia in the adult: surgical treatment and complications. Rev Med Suisse 2011;7(322):2482, 2484–8.
12. Tobin GR. Hemisoleus and reversed hemisoleus flaps. Plast Reconstr Surg 1985; 76(1):87–96.
13. Pu LIQ. Further experience with the medial hemisoleus muscle flap for soft tissue coverage of a tibial wound in the distal third of the leg. Plast Reconstr Surg 2008; 121(6):2024–8.
14. Simon SR, Mann RA, Hagy JL, et al. Role of the posterior calf muscle in normal gait. J Bone Joint Surg 1978;60A:465.
15. Zenn M, Jones G. Reconstructive surgery: anatomy, technique, and clinical application. New York: CRC Press; 2012. p. 1628–53.
16. Schierle CF, Rawlani V, Galiano RD, et al. Improving outcomes of the distally based hemisoleus flap: principles of angiosomes in flap design. Plast Reconstr Surg 2009;123(6):1748–54.
17. Thornton BP, Rosenblum WJ, Lee L. Reconstruction of limited soft-tissue defect with open tibial fracture in the distal third of the leg. Ann Plast Surg 2005;54(3): 276–80.

Distally Based Medial Hemisoleus Muscle Flap for Wound Coverage in the Distal Third of the Leg

Ahmed Ashraf Fisal, MSc[a], Mohamed Abdel-Hamid Romeih, MD[a],
Lotfy Mohamed Younes, MD[a], Mahmoud El-Rosasy, MD[b],
Pedro Rodriguez, MD[c], Michael D. Liette, DPM[d],
Suhail Masadeh, DPM[e],*

KEYWORDS

- Soleus flap • Lower limb reconstruction • Distal third tibia • Muscle flap

KEY POINTS

- Muscle flaps improve vascularity, eliminate dead space, increase collagen deposition, and increase antibiotic delivery to wound sites.
- The distally based medial hemisoleus muscle flap is a stable and reliable option for soft tissue coverage of distal third lower extremity wounds.
- The distally based medial hemisoleus flap is reliant on the distal two or three minor perforators arising from posterior tibial artery.
- The distally based medial hemisoleus flap requires a short operative time and has minimal donor site morbidity.
- The "C-point" provides a landmark to the avascular plane of flap dissection.

INTRODUCTION

The distal third of the leg is susceptible to various pathologies that require advanced soft tissue reconstruction. Open fractures, soft tissue injuries, ulcers related to diabetes, tumors, and ischemic wounds may be causative of soft tissue defects of the distal lower extremity. Management of complex soft tissue injuries in this region are

---

[a] Department of Orthopedic Surgery, Faculty of Medicine, Tanta University, Tanta University Hospital, AlGeish Street, Tanta 31511, Egypt; [b] Limb Lengthening & Reconstruction and Pediatric Orthopedics, Department of Orthopedic Surgery, Tanta University Hospital, Faculty of Medicine, Tanta University, AlGeish Street, Tanta 31511, Egypt; [c] Plastic and Reconstructive Surgery, OSF Saint Anthony Medical Center, University of Illinois, 698 Featherstone Road, Rockford, IL 61107, USA; [d] University of Cincinnati Medical Center, 231 Albert Sabin Way, ML 0513, Cincinnati, OH 45276, USA; [e] University of Cincinnati Medical Center, Cincinnati Veteran Affairs Medical Center, 231 Albert Sabin Way, ML 0513, Cincinnati, OH 45276, USA
* Corresponding author.
E-mail address: Masadesb@uc.edu

Clin Podiatr Med Surg 37 (2020) 631–647
https://doi.org/10.1016/j.cpm.2020.05.002
0891-8422/20/Published by Elsevier Inc.
podiatric.theclinics.com

challenging because of poor elasticity of the skin, the thin subcutaneous tissue covering the bone, multiple superficial tendons, and a lack of muscle bulk.[1–4] Furthermore, poor venous outflow within the area often contributes to the presence of chronic edema that can lead to venous hypertension and subsequent ulcerations. These wounds have also shown increased morbidity and high rates of osteomyelitis, frequently resulting in limb amputation.[5] Advancements in microsurgery techniques have led to the use of free tissue transfer for management of distal third defects; however, this requires a specialty center equipped to deal with the demands of the surgery and the extensive postoperative course, including constant flap monitoring.[6] Patients with severe or multiple comorbidities are often excluded from these extensive procedures and require other less invasive options.[6,7] Therefore, in small defects of the lower leg, local flaps are frequently used to provide the required soft tissue coverage.

Distally based fasciocutaneous and propeller flaps are designed to provide rapid coverage of distal lower extremity defects. They do require advanced surgical skills and specialized training, otherwise the surgeon will likely contend with a high rate of complications leading to flap failure and a larger wound. The use of fasciocutaneous flaps must be performed cautiously because they may impede the use of the underlying muscle as an alternative flap in cases of failure. The soleus muscle is frequently used for defects of the middle third of the tibia because of close proximity to the wound site and ample vascular supply. The proximally based medial hemisoleus muscle flap is rotated on its dominant pedicle to cover the midtibial region with consistent reliability, but the soleus muscle can also be used in a reverse fashion based on its distal minor pedicles to cover defects in the distal third of the lower extremity with similar outcomes.[1–4,6–11]

ANATOMY

The soleus muscle is a broad, flat muscle that is composed of a medial and lateral head with bipennate morphology.[12,13] The heads are conjoined proximally at their origin with a distinct separation distally via the intermuscular septum, otherwise known as the central raphe.[12,13] The soleus muscle is located deep to the gastrocnemius muscle within the superficial posterior compartment of the leg.[12,13] The two muscles combine as they travel distally to form the Achilles tendon near their insertion into the middle third of the calcaneus.[12,13] The origin of the soleus is broad and covers a large portion of the posterior lower leg. The lateral head of the muscle encompasses the proximal third and the posterior portion of the head of the fibula, and the medial head originates from the soleal line of the posterior tibia.[12,13] The arterial supply of medial half is via the posterior tibial artery as it branches into a dominant pedicle and three or more minor pedicles, as seen in **Fig. 1**.[12,13] The lateral head is supplied via the peroneal artery, creating independent vascularity.[12,13] Deep to the soleus muscle is a thin fascial layer that covers the tibial nerve and the posterior tibial artery as they travel to the distal medial ankle, separating the deep and superficial compartments of the leg.[12,13] The soleus, along with the gastrocnemius muscle, functions to plantarflex the ankle joint and secondarily supinate the hindfoot.[14–17] It is the synergistic action of these muscles that renders each individual component as "expendable" for use as a local muscle flap.[4,18,19]

Muscles of the lower leg have been studied extensively as sources of tissue for expedient soft tissue coverage. The understanding of the arterial supply and the orientation of the vascular pedicles allows for muscle transfer while maintaining intact perfusion and viability.[10] Mathes and Nahai[14–17] developed a classification system recognizing five basic patterns of muscle circulation. This classification identifies

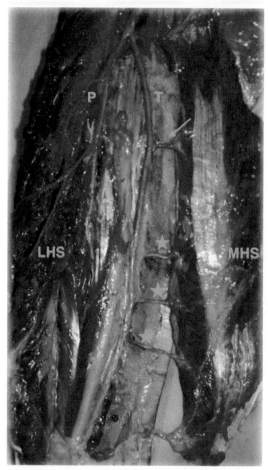

Fig. 1. Demonstration of the medial (MHS) and lateral (LHS) hemisoleus muscles and their accompanying vascularity. The LHS is supplied by the peroneal (P) artery and the MHS is supplied by the posterior tibial (T) artery. The dominant proximal pedicle to the MHS is shown with an *arrow* and the distal minor pedicles are shown with *stars*. (*Courtesy of* S. Masadeh DPM, Cincinnati, OH.)

vascular pedicles (artery and its two venae comitantes surrounded by a cuff of adventitia) entry point, number, and size, which influence the choice and potential use of a muscle as a flap.[10,14–17] Pedicles are divided into either dominant or minor, with dominant pedicles capable of nourishing the entire muscle independently after ligation of the minor pedicles and muscle transposition.[10,12,14–17] If the pedicle is only able to sustain a small portion of the muscle, it is termed a minor pedicle.[10,14–17] These minor pedicles communicate via the internal architecture of the muscle, as compared with segmental pedicles, which supply only a specific segment of a muscle without internal communications. These intramuscular communications allow for larger areas of muscle to be transposed and maintain adequate perfusion. When the arterial supply of a muscle consists of a dominant pedicle and multiple minor pedicles, it is classified as a type II muscle, the predominant type found within the lower extremity.[14–17]

The dominant pedicles have shown little variability in number and location, whereas minor pedicles are often variable in both categories.[10,14–17] In the lower extremity, the dominant pedicle enters the muscle close to the origin, and therefore the arc of rotation for the muscle transposition occurs in a proximally based direction.[10] The soleus muscle is commonly used in a "standard fashion," or designed on its dominant pedicle, for defects in the middle third of the lower extremity. When the dominant pedicle is ligated, and the flap is sustained entirely by the distal minor pedicles, it is defined as a "reverse" flap. A minor pedicle can reliably sustain a specific segment of the muscle but is not able to sustain the entire muscle exclusively.[10,12] When maintaining multiple minor pedicles, the blood supply remains orthogonal aided by an axial vessel often termed "the main drag."[10,12] Together, these minor pedicles can supply the muscle and allow for a reverse or turnover flap with a distally based arc of rotation.

SURGICAL TECHNIQUE

The initial steps of the surgical technique are similar to that of the proximally based medial hemisoleus flap. The patient is placed in the supine position with a bump under the contralateral side to allow for external rotation of the extremity. The medial boarder of the tibia is identified and the cleavage point between the gastrocnemius and soleus muscles is located, which typically occurs 2 to 3 cm distal from the tibial tuberosity. Next, the incision line is outlined from the proximal tibia to the level of the medial malleolus. The distal perforators are identified with a handheld Doppler and their locations are mapped on the extremity. In addition, thermal imaging may be useful to identify "hot spots" that correspond to perforators and aid in more reliable perforator mapping, as seen in **Fig. 2**.[20] This may be evaluated and determined by performing a preoperative angiogram or computed tomography angiography if necessary.[21] The incision is then made through the skin and subcutaneous fascia, starting proximally from the junction between the proximal and middle one-third of the tibia, and stopped distally, approximately 6 cm proximal to the medial malleolus. The incision is deepened to the level of the deep fascia, and the great saphenous vein and the saphenous nerve are identified and protected. The deep fascia is then incised to identify and isolate the gastrocnemius muscle, and the fasciotomy is continued distally. The minor perforators are more superficial within the distal third of the lower extremity and care must be taken to avoid injury during dissection. The plantaris tendon is located between the gastrocnemius and the soleus muscle and can serve as an anatomic landmark to ensure identification of the proper plane of dissection as seen in **Fig. 3**.

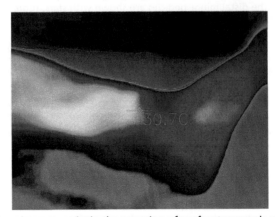

Fig. 2. Thermal imaging may assist in the mapping of perforator vessels preoperatively and aiding in more successful flap design. (*Courtesy of* S. Masadeh DPM, Cincinnati, OH.)

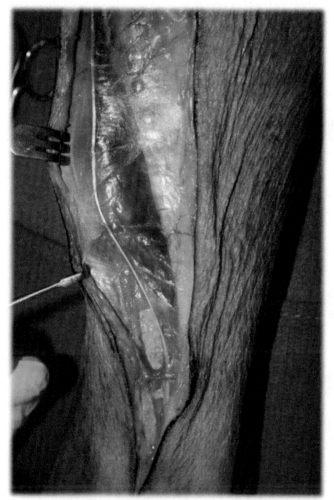

Fig. 3. Identification of the plantaris tendon within the superficial posterior compartment between the gastrocnemius and the soleus muscles. (*Courtesy of* S. Masadeh DPM, Cincinnati, OH.)

The gastrocnemius muscle is then gently reflected superior and lateral and separated from the soleus muscle as seen in **Fig. 4**. The plane between the gastrocnemius and soleus is often referred to as "avascular"; however, there are direct muscular arterial branches that need to be identified and ligated when necessary during dissection. The gastrocnemius muscle is elevated past the central raphe of the soleus and the dissection is carried from proximal to distal until the conjoined tendon of the Achilles is reached (**Fig. 5**). Most authors recommend detachment of the soleus muscle fibers from the tibia to identify the posterior tibial artery and its perforators, but we maintain the soleus attachment to the tibia during flap elevation to allow for traction and countertraction. This facilitates easier dissection of the distal soleus from the Achilles tendon and assists in preserving the aponeurosis of the tendon.

As the soleus curves from its fibrous attachment to the tibia, it leads to a distinct dissection plane that the senior author (P.R.) has termed the "C-point," as seen in **Fig. 6**. The "C-point" is an avascular zone that allows for atraumatic separation of the soleus muscle and the fascia of the deep posterior compartment. Dissection in this zone provides a safe place of dissection that allows protection during dissection to the thin fascial layer overlying the tibial neurovascular bundle, separating the superficial from the deep posterior leg compartments (**Fig. 7**). The "C point" also serves as a reliable landmark for the first "large" minor pedicle to the distal medial hemisoleus. This perforator has the largest caliber of the minor perforators and serves as the ideal pivot point for the flap, if it allows for enough arc of rotation to cover the soft tissue deficit. Typically, there are two to three additional minor perforators of a smaller caliber that may further aid in flap perfusion.[1–4,6,7,10,12] It is critical for success to preserve as many of these distal perforators as possible to improve flap survivability while allowing enough flap rotation to reach the defect.

Once the soleus muscle is elevated proximally at the "C-point," the tibial attachment is transected and the major and minor pedicles are identified. The muscle is then transected proximally in a transverse direction past the soleus midline. The intermuscular septum/central-raphe that separates the medial and later heads is more visible on the deep surface of the muscle but is also readily palpable during dissection. The muscle is then split longitudinally, just lateral to the central raphe, preserving the

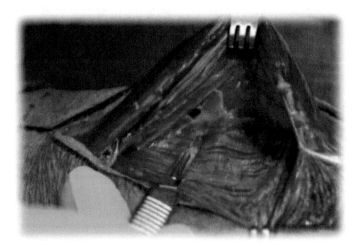

Fig. 4. Separation of the gastrocnemius muscle from the underlying soleus muscle. (*Courtesy of* S. Masadeh DPM, Cincinnati, OH.)

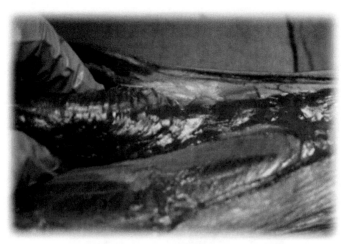

Fig. 5. Separation of the gastrocnemius muscle from the soleus muscle as they join to form the Achilles tendon. The soleus muscle is separated without disturbing the tendon or the peritendinous structures. (*Courtesy of* S. Masadeh DPM, Cincinnati, OH.)

intermuscular nutrient artery within the now elevated medial hemisoleus flap as seen in **Fig. 8.** This further assists in arterial perfusion through the communicating vessels from the peroneal artery and increases the reliability of the distally based flap (**Fig. 9**). The muscle is then rotated and inset into the defect without tension so as to minimize postoperative complications. Tunneling of the flap is not recommended because this can cause venous congestion.[21,22] If additional flap excursion is needed, the muscle epimysium is scored or removed to allow for expansion of the muscle and improve the reach. Intraoperative acoustic Doppler is then used to evaluate the perforator and to ensure that kinking of the pedicle has not occurred. At this point, the muscle can be covered with a split-thickness skin graft or temporized with a dermal regenerative template. A drain is then placed between the superficial and deep posterior compartments at the harvest site to allow for postoperative fluid management. The donor site is closed primarily, and the limb is immobilized; this entire process is summarized in **Figs. 10–13**.

POSTOPERATIVE CARE

Postoperatively, the patient is placed on a strict bed rest protocol with leg elevation and appropriate anticoagulation therapy for 1 week. The drain is removed when fluid output is less than 30 mL per 24-hour period. After the first postoperative week, the patient can place the limb in dependency at increasing intervals, typically 15-minute sessions, three times a day. The dependency interval is increased by 15 minutes daily for the remainder of postoperative Week 2. If extensive edema is noted, then the elevation protocol is set back to the previous days timing until the edema subsides. We recommend compression stockings 20 to 30 mm Hg for 1 year postoperatively for edema management and to assist in flap remodeling. Weight bearing is initiated at Week 3, pending osseous stability or other appropriate management of any associated fractures.

ANALYSIS/DISCUSSION

Coverage of soft tissue defects in the distal third of the leg is challenging and often associated with long-term morbidity.[1–4] The refinement and success of microsurgical

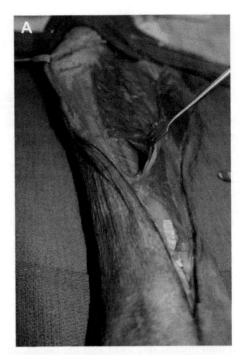

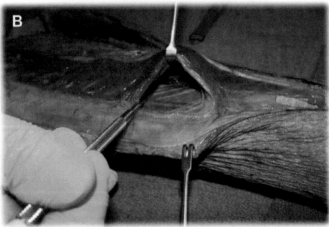

Fig. 6. (*A, B*) Relative avascular zone termed the "C-Point," which serves as the anatomic location to separate the soleus muscle from the thin fascial layer separating the deep posterior compartment from the superficial posterior compartment of the lower leg. (*Courtesy of* S. Masadeh DPM, Cincinnati, OH.)

techniques has largely replaced the use of local flaps for the management of these defects. However, microsurgeons may not be readily available to provide support for these challenging cases and not all hospitals are equipped to handle this type of complex reconstructive surgery.[6,7] As understanding of the vascular supply of muscles and their clinical applications has improved, the use of local muscle transposition as definitive treatments has additionally improved. The key to limb preservation in soft tissue loss of the distal lower extremity is early and reliable coverage. To address the

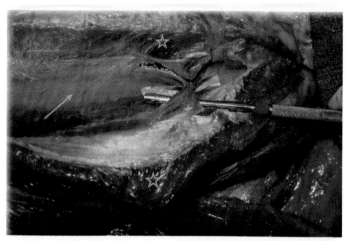

Fig. 7. Proximal dominant perforator to the medial hemisoleus is identified by the freer. The flexor digitorum longus (*superior star*), the thin fascia (*arrow*) overlying the neurovascular bundle, separating the superficial and deep posterior compartments of the lower extremity, and the medial hemisoleus (*bottom star*) are identified as landmarks. (*Courtesy of* S. Masadeh DPM, Cincinnati, OH.)

increasing need for the management of this type of defect, various local and reginal options, such as cross leg flaps, reverse fasciocutaneous flaps, and propeller flaps for wound coverage, have been described, each with its own risks and benefits.

Muscle flaps provide an excellent coverage option and historically have been regarded as immunologically superior in contaminated wounds. They are versatile, malleable, and have demonstrated the ability to effectively fill dead space while facilitating antibiotic delivery to the wound.[23–26] Muscle flaps have also demonstrated an increase in the rates of collagen deposition and tissue ingrowth at the wound site.[23–26] Gosain and colleagues,[25] in a canine inoculation experimental model, established a rapid decline in bacterial wound count within the first 24 hours after muscle flap application. They postulated that the muscle surface and blood flow

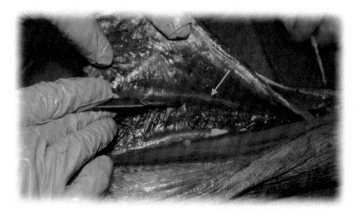

Fig. 8. Splitting the muscle longitudinally lateral to the central raphe to include the nutrient artery with the medial hemisoleus flap. The arrow is pointing to the central raphe. (*Courtesy of* S. Masadeh DPM, Cincinnati, OH.)

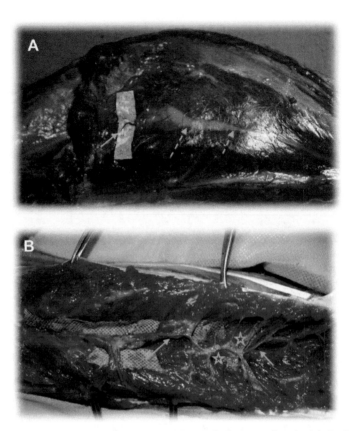

Fig. 9. (*A, B*) The nutrient artery (*solid arrows*) beneath the central raphe (*dashed arrows*) is identified, assisting in the perfusion of the flap with contributions from the peroneal artery and the internal muscular communicating arterial branches (*stars*). (*Courtesy of* S. Masadeh DPM, Cincinnati, OH.)

properties allowed for rapid tissue ingrowth, giving the muscle tissue superiority in bacterial suppression.[25] Recent literature has debated the efficacy of muscle flaps versus fasciocutaneous flaps and their use in infected wound beds.[27–30] Both types of flap composition have shown comparable outcomes in terms of limb salvage, but muscle flaps often experience lower rates of venous congestion.[22,27–31] Regardless of the type of flap used and their ability to inhibit bacterial growth, wound preparation and osseous stabilization are the cornerstone for successful outcomes. Any type of flap is destined to fail if the wound bed is inadequately prepared and the underlying osseous structure is unstable. In addition, poor wound bed preparation alters flap neovascularization leading to a permanently pedicle dependent flap.[32] Selection of either flap should be based on the patients' reconstructive need and the size of defect.[31]

The soleus muscle flap, as first described by Tobin[33] in 1985, is used mostly for tissue loss in the middle third of the tibia, which is based on its dominant pedicle. The distally based medial hemisoleus muscle flap, however, relies on the distal most two to three minor pedicles.[1–4,6,7,10] When using the soleus in a distal fashion, there is a potential decrease in flap reliability, because the minor pedicles may not supply a large segment of the muscle. However, the intramuscular arterial territories spanned

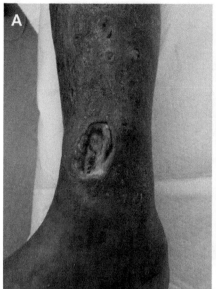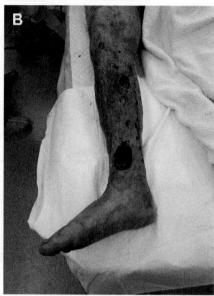

Fig. 10. (*A, B*) Predebridement and postdebridement of the wound site in preparation for eventual distally based medially hemisoleus coverage. Visible is exposed bone throughout the distal most wound. (*Courtesy of* S. Masadeh DPM, Cincinnati, OH.)

by these distal perforators are linked within via small-caliber choke vessels that allow bidirectional flow of blood.[12] By maintaining multiple distal perforators, the flap can capture more choke vessels and improve viability. Additionally, the soleus muscle with its medial and lateral heads receives dual blood supply from the posterior tibial artery and peroneal artery, respectively. Fayman and colleagues[34] has shown in barium angiographic studies the presence of significant vascular communications between these two systems via a distinct intermuscular septum. This T-shape intramuscular septum provides a site of separation of the distal half of the muscle. By modifying the flap harvest technique and preserving the intermuscular septum, the flap has additional blood supply from the peroneal system through the lateral half of the muscle, providing additional perfusion support.

As is the case with performing any limb salvage surgery, careful patient selection and preoperative planning is paramount for success. Computed tomography angiography and color duplex ultrasound assist in the preoperative identification of muscular perforators to ensure their inclusion.[11,20,35–37] Furthermore, duplex Doppler scans aid in the assessment of the velocity of arterial flow. Hong and colleagues[38] demonstrated greater success in free flaps when the recipient artery had a velocity greater than 15 to 20 cm/s. To our knowledge, optimal perforator velocity for muscle flaps, specifically distally based hemisoleus, has not been established. A handheld audible Doppler allows for rapid perforator identification but does not provide information about the caliber or the velocity of the vessel. According to Houdek and colleagues,[21] the caliber of the distal arterial perforator should be a minimum of 1 mm and the venae comitantes 1.5 mm or greater in diameter for improved venous outflow. The use of MRI to preoperatively determine adequate muscle size is not necessary unless there is significant atrophy of the leg.[39] In all patients with ulcers related to diabetes, strict control of blood glucose and adequate nutrition are prerequisites to surgery. In patients who sustained traumatic wounds with underlying fractures, it is critical to assess viability

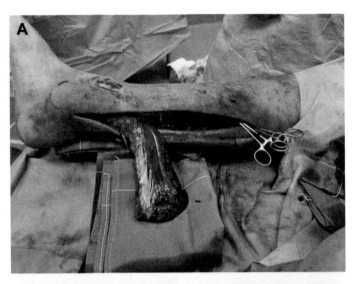

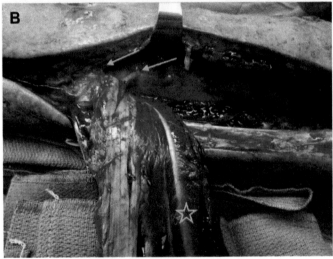

Fig. 11. (*A, B*) Elevation of the medial hemisoleus muscle with intact central raphe (*star*) and identifiable distal perforators (*arrows*). (*Courtesy of* S. Masadeh DPM, Cincinnati, OH.)

of the muscle and the distal perforators within the zone of injury, because damage to the muscle or the perforators may preclude the use of this flap.[11] This flap use should be cautiously approached in patients that are heavy smokers because they face a greater risk of partial flap necrosis and other postoperative complications.[1–4,9]

Potential complications of the distally based medial hemisoleus flap include partial or complete flap necrosis. Complete flap necrosis is rare and is usually caused by damage to the pedicle or considerable damage to the muscle at the time of initial injury.[21] When partial necrosis occurs, it is typically at the distal margin and is often debrided with or without muscle readvancement, pending exposure of vital structures or retained hardware. In a series of 10 patients, Pu[4] reported distal flap necrosis in two patients, or 20% distal flap necrosis in defects ranging from 9 to 60 cm^2.

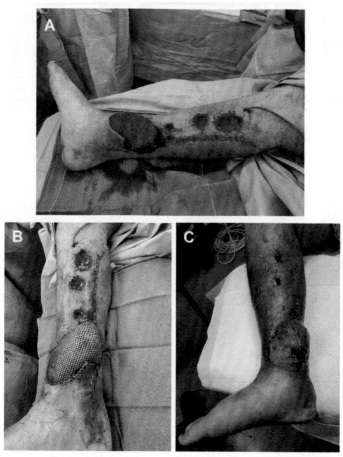

Fig. 12. (*A*) Rotation and tension-free inset of the medial hemisoleus flap and drain application for fluid management. (*B*) Split-thickness skin graft application. (*C*) Final end product fully healed. (*Courtesy of* S. Masadeh DPM, Cincinnati, OH.)

Rabbani and colleagues[9] reported on 37 cases treated with a distally based medial hemisoleus. In their series three (8.1%) cases had partial flap necrosis and one patient with partial necrosis with dehiscence (2.7%) requiring reoperation. They concluded that the flap is reliable in wounds without muscle trauma and limited defect size to less than 50 cm^2.[9] Houdek and colleagues[21] reported on 10 cases; four patients required debridement and repeat skin grafting with one patient requiring flap advancement. Kauffman and colleagues[7] reported on 12 cases of soleus flap coverage of distal third tibial defects where they had 75% limb salvage rates. However, in their series, one patient experienced complete flap loss and two of the patients required below-knee amputations.[7] Furthermore, 66% of the patients had at least one postoperative complication.[7] They concluded that trauma, smoking, radiation, and peripheral vascular occlusive disease should be considered relative contraindications to the use of the medial hemisoleus flap in the distal third of the leg.[7] In our clinical experience, we have encountered partial flap loss requiring debridement and skin grafting. Although several publications advocate a single-stage procedure, we opt for flap temporization with a dermal regenerative template

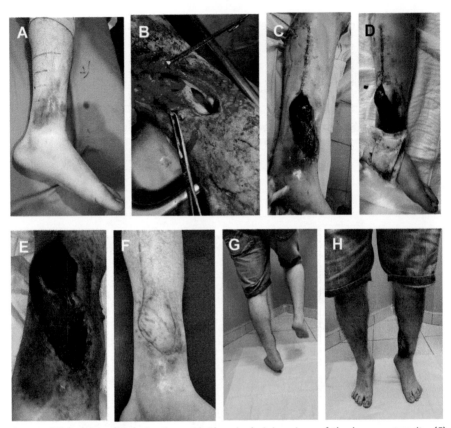

Fig. 13. (*A*) Preoperative evaluation with chronic draining sinus of the lower extremity. (*B*) Initial debridement to healthy bleeding margins with a positive "paprika sign" of the exposed tibia. (*C*) Inset and rotation of the medial hemisoleus muscle flap. (*D*) Temporizing of the muscle flap site with a bilayer dermal regenerative template to reduce adhesions and facilitate eventual split-thickness skin graft. (*E*) Muscle flap with neodermis after dermal regenerative template. (*F*) Healed soft tissue deficit of the lower extremity. (*G, H*) No loss of function of plantarflexion strength because of the preservation of the lateral head of the soleus muscle and the gastrocnemius muscle. (*Courtesy of* S. Masadeh DPM, Cincinnati, OH.)

for 7 to 14 days. This improves flap survivability and creates a neodermis over the exposed muscle, preventing adherence of the split-thickness skin graft to the muscle and minimizes shearing forces and failures. The temporization additionally improves split-thickness skin graft because it creates a highly vascularized wound bed that readily provides the nutrients for the early stages of split-thickness skin graft incorporation.

In conclusion, the distally based medial hemisoleus flaps provides reliable coverage of soft tissue defects in the distal third of the lower extremity. This flap does not require microvascular anastomosis and has proven to provide reliable coverage in defects of the distal leg while serving as an alternative to free flap reconstruction.[8]

CLINICAL CARE POINTS

- The distally based medial hemisoleus flap provides a reliable coverage option for defects of the distal third of the lower extremity.

- Harvesting half of the muscle, and preserving the lateral hemisoleus, retains ankle plantarflexion strength.
- The medial hemisoleus has a consistent blood supply including dominant and minor pedicles with improved arc of rotation.
- Careful patient selection and preoperative planning is critical for a successful hemisoleus flap.
- Wound bed preparation and osseous stability are the cornerstone for successful soft tissue reconstruction.
- Incorporating the midline raphe with the muscle flap, preserving the distal perforators, and delaying split-thickness skin graft may improve flap outcome.

DISCLOSURE

The authors have nothing to disclose.

REFERENCES

1. Pu LIQ. Further experience with the medial hemisoleus muscle flap for soft tissue coverage of a tibial wound in the distal third of the leg. Plast Reconstr Surg 2008; 121(6):2024–8.
2. Pu LL. Soft-tissue reconstruction of an open tibial wound in the distal third of the leg: a new treatment algorithm. Ann Plast Surg 2007;58(1):78–83.
3. Pu LL. Successful soft-tissue coverage of a tibial wound in the distal third of the leg with a medial hemisoleus muscle flap. Plast Reconstr Surg 2005;115(1): 245–51.
4. Pu LLQ. The reversed medial hemisoleus muscle flap and its role in reconstruction of an open tibial wound in the lower third of the leg. Ann Plast Surg 2006;56: 59–64.
5. Faglia E, Clerici G, Caminiti M, et al. Influence of osteomyelitis location in the foot of diabetic patients with transtibial amputation. Foot Ankle Int 2013;34(2):222–7.
6. Thornton BP, Rosenblum WJ, Lee L. Reconstruction of limited soft-tissue defect with open tibial fracture in the distal third of the leg. Ann Plast Surg 2005;54(3): 276–80.
7. Kauffman CA, Lahoda LU, Cederna PS, et al. Use of soleus muscle flaps for coverage of distal third tibial defects. J Reconstr Microsurg 2004;20(8):593–7.
8. Nazneen A, Sarkar A. Distally based medial hemi-soleus muscle flap for coverage in the distal third of the leg. IOSR Journal of Dental and Medical Sciences 2019;18(5):49–53.
9. Rabbani MJ, Ata-ul-Haq, Riaz A, et al. Distally based medial hemisoleus flap: reliable option for distal tibial wounds. J Coll Physicians Surg Pak 2018;28(2): 129–32.
10. Thorne CH, Chung KC, Gosain AK, et al. Grabb and Smith's plastic surgery. 7th edition. Philadelphia: Wolters Kluwer Health Adis (ESP); 2013.
11. Zenn M, Jones G. Reconstructive surgery: anatomy, technique, and clinical application. New York: CRC Press; 2012. p. 1628–53.
12. Raveendran SS, Kumaragama KGJL. Arterial supply of the soleus muscle: anatomical study of fifty lower limbs. Clin Anat 2003;16:248–52.
13. Kelikian AS, Sarrafian SK. Sarrafians anatomy of the foot and ankle, 3rd edition. Philadelphia: Lippincott Williams & Wilkins. p. 326–36.
14. Mathes SJ, Nahai F. Classification of the vascular anatomy of muscle: experimental and clinical correlation. Plast Reconstr Surg 1981;67:177–87.

15. Mathes SJ, Nahai F. Clinical applications for muscle and musculocutaneous flaps. St Louis (MO): CV Mosby; 1982. p. 27–9.
16. Mathes SJ, Nahai F. Muscle flap transposition with function preservation: technical and clinical considerations. Plast Reconstr Surg 1980;66:242–9.
17. Mathes SJ, Nahai F. Reconstructive surgery: principles, anatomy, and technique. New York: Churchill Livingstone; 1997.
18. Hallock GG. Getting the most from the soleus muscle. Ann Plast Surg 1996;36: 139–46.
19. Simon SR, Mann RA, Hagy JL, et al. Role of the posterior calf muscle in normal gait. J Bone Joint Surg 1978;60A:465.
20. Hallock GG. Doppler sonography and color duplex imaging for planning a perforator flap. Clin Plast Surg 2003;30:347–57.
21. Houdek MT, Wagner ER, Wyles CC, et al. Reverse medial hemisoleus flaps for coverage of distal third leg wounds: a technical trick. J Orthop Trauma 2016; 30(4):138–42.
22. De Souza Filho MV, De Oliveira Teixeira JC, De Castro OC. Reversed hemisoleus flap for wound coverage in the distal third of the leg: retalho hemissolear reverso na reconstrução de defeito do terço distal da perna. Rev Col Bras Cir 2011;26(4): 710–3.
23. Calderon W, Chang N, Mathes SJ. Comparison of the effect of bacterial inoculation in musculocutaneous and fasciocutaneous flaps. Plast Reconstr Surg 1986; 77(5):785–94.
24. Chang N, Mathes SJ. Comparison of the effect of bacterial inoculation in musculocutaneous and random-pattern flaps. Plast Reconstr Surg 1982;70(1):1–10.
25. Gosain A, Chang N, Mathes S, et al. A study of the relationship between blood flow and bacterial inoculation in musculocutaneous and fasciocutaneous flaps. Plast Reconstr Surg 1990;86(6):1152–63.
26. Klebuc M, Menn Z. Muscle flaps and their role in limb salvage. Methodist DeBakey Cardiovasc J 2013;9(2):95–9.
27. Hallock GG. The utility of both muscle and fascia flaps in severe upper extremity trauma. J Trauma 2002;53:61–5.
28. Mathes SJ, Alpert BS, Chang N. Use of the muscle flap in chronic osteomyelitis: experimental and clinical correlation. Plast Reconstr Surg 1982;69(5):815–29.
29. Salgado CJ, Mardini S, Jamali AA, et al. Muscle versus nonmuscle flaps in the reconstruction of chronic osteomyelitis defects. Plast Reconstr Surg 2006; 118(6):1401–11.
30. Yazar S, Lin CH, Lin YT, et al. Outcome comparison between free muscle and free fasciocutaneous flaps for reconstruction of distal third and ankle traumatic open tibial fractures. Plast Reconstr Surg 2006;117(7):2468–75.
31. Cho EH, Shammas RL, Carney MJ, et al. Muscle versus fasciocutaneous free flaps in lower extremity traumatic reconstruction: a multicenter outcomes analysis. Plast Reconstr Surg 2018;141(1):191–9.
32. Millican PG, Poole MD. Peripheral neovascularization of muscle and musculocutaneous flaps. Br J Plast Surg 1985;38:369–74.
33. Tobin GR. Hemisoleus and reversed hemisoleus flaps. Plast Reconstr Surg 1985; 76(1):87–96.
34. Fayman MS, Orak F, Hugo B, et al. The distally based split soleus muscle flap. Br J Plast Surg 1987;40:20–6.
35. Blondeel PN, Beyens G, Verhaeghe R, et al. Doppler flowmetry in the planning of perforator flaps. Br J Plast Surg 1998;51(3):202–9.

36. Giunta RE, Geisweid A, Feller AM. The value of preoperative Doppler sonography for planning free perforator flaps. Plast Reconstr Surg 2000;105(7):2381–6.
37. Khan UD, Miller JG. Reliability of handheld Doppler in planning local perforator–based flaps for extremities. Aesthetic Plast Surg 2007;31(5):521–5.
38. Suh HS, Oh TS, Lee HS, et al. A new approach for reconstruction of diabetic foot wounds using the angiosome and supermicrosurgery concept. Plast Reconstr Surg 2016;138(4):702–9.
39. Attinger CE, Clemens MW, Ducic I, et al. The use of local muscle flaps in foot and ankle reconstruction. In: Dockery GD, Crawford ME, editors. Lower Extremity Soft Tissue & Cutaneous Plastic Surgery. 2nd edition. Philadelphia: Elsevier Ltd. W.B. Saunders; 2012. p. 269–88.

Lower Limb Muscle Flaps
The Reverse Peroneus Brevis Flap

Phuoc V. Bui, DPM[a,1], Dominic A. Rizzo, DPM[a,b],*

KEYWORDS

- Peroneus brevis flap • Muscle flap • Lower leg and hindfoot reconstruction
- Wound coverage • Limb salvage

KEY POINTS

- The peroneus brevis flap is classified as a type IV muscle, meaning it has no dominant pedicles but has instead segmental vascular pedicles.
- The peroneus brevis muscle flap is able to cover small to medium-sized defects that can have exposed bone, tendon, or both. It can be an excellent alternative to more difficult procedures, such as free flaps.
- This muscle flap also can be used for the following: for failed/revisional Charcot, to enhance arthrodesis, and to treat osteomyelitis by increasing vascularity and local antibiotic delivery.
- It is an excellent alternative to fasciocutaneous, adipofascial, or free flaps in covering chronic soft tissue defects in the lower extremity.

INTRODUCTION

Chronic ulcerations of the lower extremity are common, complex, and very difficult to treat owing to the multiple etiologies and comorbidities associated with them.[1–5] Soft tissue defects that are centered around the distal lower leg with exposed bone or tendons present lower extremity surgeons little to work with: lateral malleolus, Achilles tendon, plantar calcaneus, and dorsum of the foot. The peroneus brevis (PB) muscle flap is readily available to cover small to medium-sized defects at these areas.[6,7]

The longer a wound is open, the more the risk for infection, amputation, morbidity, mortality, and increased health care dollars. Despite advances in wound care modalities, the soft tissue reconstructive surgeon still needs to follow an algorithm that addresses a wound problem from simple to complex.[8,9] The end goal of any open wound is closure of that wound, and the coverage options available include local wound care

[a] Department of Podiatric Surgery, TriHealth – Bethesda North Hospital, Montgomery, OH, USA; [b] Cincinnati Lower Extremity Reconstructive Institute, Foot and Ankle Specialists of Cincinnati
[1] Present address: 2634 Fernview Court, Cincinnati, OH 45212.
* Corresponding author. 4260 Glendale Milford Road, Unit 103, Blue Ash, OH 45242.
E-mail address: rizzodpm@gmail.com

Clin Podiatr Med Surg 37 (2020) 649–670
https://doi.org/10.1016/j.cpm.2020.07.004
0891-8422/20/© 2020 Elsevier Inc. All rights reserved.

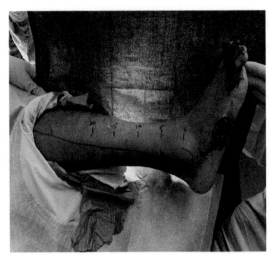

Fig. 1. The typical skin incision for the PB flap, showing the perforators mapped out, each at 5-cm increments.

products, negative-pressure wound therapy (NPWT), and split-thickness skin grafts (STSGs).[5,8] When these complex soft tissue defects fail to heal by conventional treatments, immediate wound coverage options are available, including local cutaneous flaps, fasciocutaneous or adipofascial flaps, muscle flaps, and free flaps.[5,7,9–11] The evolution of orthoplastics and microsurgery has greatly expanded the armamentarium of the lower extremity reconstructive surgeon to manage even the most complex soft tissue defects.[12]

Local cutaneous flaps are able to cover soft tissue defects readily and with minor donor morbidity. Disadvantages, however, are that they have a limited arc of rotation

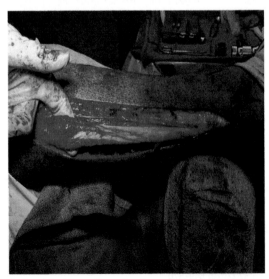

Fig. 2. Once through the skin, blunt dissection is used to separate the peroneus longus from the PB muscle bellies.

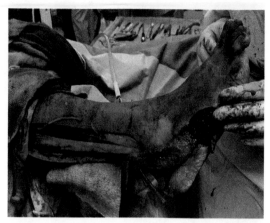

Fig. 3. The 180° rotation of the harvested muscle flap onto the defect.

and limited amount of tissue coverage and that distal flap necrosis is common. An advantage is that they have lower complication rates compared with free flaps.[1,4,7–9,11]

Adipofascial flaps are amenable to covering small to moderate-sized defects due to their versatility, simplicity, limited donor site morbidity, and minimized risk of injury to major neurovascular structures.[8,13–15] As pedicled flaps, there is no distant donor site morbidity because they can be closed primarily, have minimal sensory loss, and leave a cosmetically acceptable scar.[15,16]

Muscle flaps are better able to conform to 3-dimensional wounds, fill dead spaces, and decrease risk of infection by improving vascularity and antibiotic delivery, rapid collagen deposition, tissue regeneration, and preservation of limb length, thus making them a first-line choice when dealing with those issues.[3,5,7,9,11,17–19]

Free flaps also have been reported to have failure rates as high as 33%.[5,20] Free flaps are technically demanding and difficult, have prolonged operative time and costs, have donor site morbidity, have increased muscle bulk, and require sophisticated equipment and a well-trained surgical team.[5,7–9,11,19,21,22]

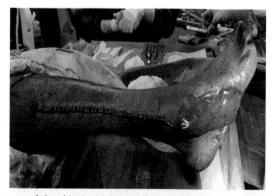

Fig. 4. Primary closure of the skin incision usually is attainable. Here, the bilayer skin substitute is applied on top of the muscle flap and secured in place with nonabsorbable sutures.

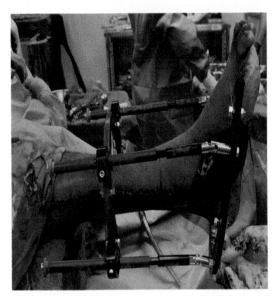

Fig. 5. This muscle flap usually needs to be immobilized and offloaded with a static external fixator, especially if it crosses the ankle joint.

The PB flap contains a dense web of intramuscular vascular connections between the perforators of the anterior tibial and peroneal arteries proximally and only from the peroneal artery distally. Also, distally, retrograde flow is provided from the posterior tibial artery.[23–25] This flap commonly is chosen by the lower extremity reconstructive surgeon due to its ease and quick elevation, safety, constant vascularity, manageable donor site morbidity, and, last but not least, reliability of soft tissue coverage over bone and tendons. The PB flap provides enough coverage for small to moderate-sized defects of the lower extremity.[3,8,21,26,27]

The article serves as a review regarding the utility of the PB muscle flap in reconstructing complex lower extremity ulcerations recalcitrant to advanced wound care modalities and its application in treating pathologic fractures, osteomyelitis (OM), and failed Charcot revisions for limb salvage purposes.

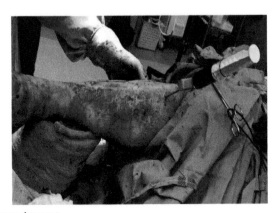

Fig. 6. Bone marrow harvest.

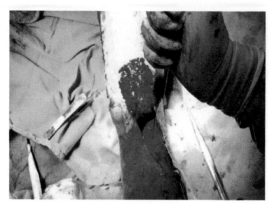

Fig. 7. Injecting of spun-down BMAC and PRP onto done site and muscle flap.

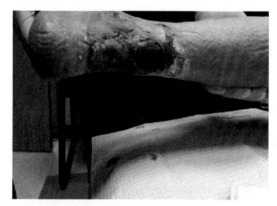

Fig. 8. A 2-year-old chronic posterior Achilles wound.

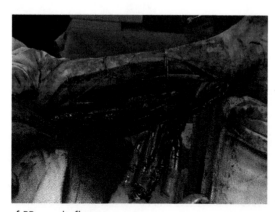

Fig. 9. Harvesting of PB muscle flap.

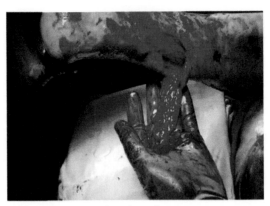

Fig. 10. Subcutaneous tunnel to posterior ulceration.

HISTORY

The PB muscle flap's blood supply has been well established by Mathes and Nahai in 1981,[25] when they originally classified it as type II, meaning it had 1 dominant pedicle and many minor pedicles.[25] It later was reclassified as type IV, which meant it has no dominant pedicles but instead segmented vascular pedicles. This was confirmed via cadaver dissection.[8,28] The first time the distally based pedicle PB muscle flap was described was in 2001, showing that it was a good choice to cover defects at the lateral and medial malleolus and distal Achilles tendon region. It also helped eliminate deep defects where exposures of osteosynthesis material, bone, or tendons were present.[26]

ANATOMY

The PB muscle is a bipennate muscle that originates from the distal two-thirds on the lateral surface of the fibula. Its tendon lies deep and anterior to the peroneus longus at the level of the lateral malleolus and inserts at the base of the fifth metatarsal to function in eversion of the foot.[11] It is innervated by the superficial peroneal nerve (SPN), and its blood supply proximally is by perforators from the anterior tibial artery that

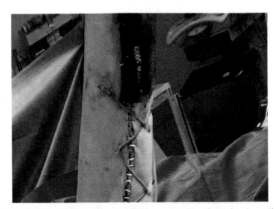

Fig. 11. Covered bilayer skin substitute and PB harvest site closed primarily with staples and vessel loops to decreased skin tension.

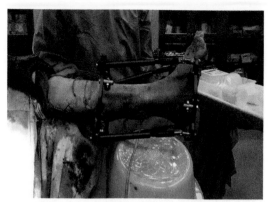

Fig. 12. NPWT and application of static circular external fixator.

enter through the anterior intermuscular septum, while distally, it is by perforators from the peroneal artery that enter through the posterior intermuscular septum, making up the pedicles.[29] This has been shown and demonstrated in cadaveric studies, which show that, on average, the muscle has 5 pedicles, with the most distal pedicle approximately 4.3 cm from the tip of the lateral malleolus. The average maximum width of the muscle was between 2.8 cm and 3.3 cm and the average length was between 21 cm and 25 cm.[8,11]

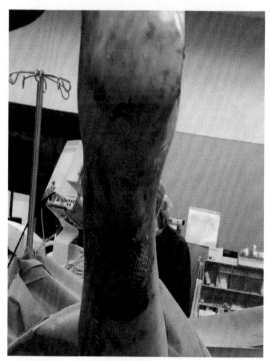

Fig. 13. STSG 4 weeks later.

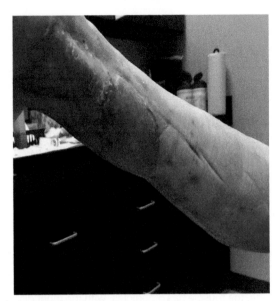

Fig. 14. Fully healed 14 weeks.

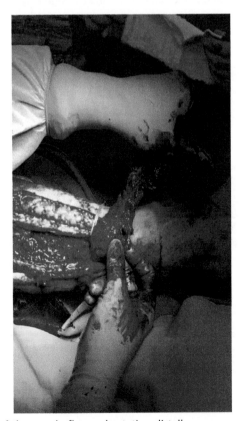

Fig. 15. Harvesting of the muscle flap and rotating distally.

Eren and colleagues[26] have shown that the blood supply of the distally based pedicle PB muscle flap received retrograde perfusion from the posterior tibial artery and antegrade perfusion from the peroneal artery. Although during flap harvest, the proximal pedicles of either the anterior tibial or peroneal arteries are sacrificed, only preserving the attachment of the muscle to the distal 6 cm of the fibula is needed to maintain adequate blood supply.[8,26] So, for cases of the PB muscle flap employed, make sure to check the patency of the peroneal artery and its runoff distally past the ankle joint for better chance of success.[8]

SURGICAL TECHNIQUE
Peroneus Brevis Muscle Flap Harvest

- Patient is supine on the operating table with a bump under the ipsilateral hip.
- No tourniquet is used.
- Anatomic dissection, electrocautery, and hydrogen peroxide are used for hemostasis. Alternatively, platelet-poor plasma from bone marrow harvest can be used.
- The 5-6 perforators are mapped out via Doppler and marked, which helps for planning purposes when applying the external fixator in addition to knowing the pivot point with the muscle flap.
- Skin incision is outlined as follows: parallel and 1 cm posterior to the fibula (but alternatively it can be in line with the fibula); proximally, it starts 3 cm distal to the

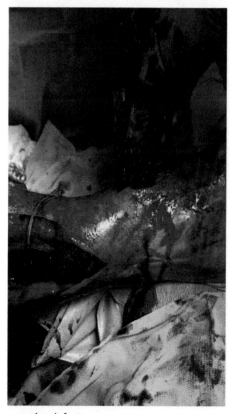

Fig. 16. Tunneling to cover the defect.

fibular head; and distally, it ends 5 cm to 6 cm proximal to the tip of the fibula (**Fig. 1**).
- This incision placement is best to avoid the common peroneal nerve proximally and both the SPN and sural nerves distally.
- After incision, once finished with the subcutaneous and adipose layers, identify the deep fascia and expose the peroneal compartment via a fasciotomy.
- Identify and protect the SPN, which is superior to the peroneal tendons.
- Blunt dissection is performed to separate the peroneus longus from the PB muscle belly (**Fig. 2**).
- Transect the PB muscle at its most proximal attachment, making sure to avoid the common peroneal nerve.
- As the brevis muscle flap is harvested, check perfusion via bleeding with bulldog clamps because this allows determining if the most proximal perforators can be sacrificed.
- Apply the bone marrow aspirate concentrate (BMAC) and platelet-rich plasma (PRP) (as discussed later) to the wound bed before placement of the muscle flap.
- Rotate the muscle flap 180o and inset into the soft tissue defect distally either through a skin incision or a subcutaneous tunnel and loosely suture in place with absorbable sutures (**Fig. 3**).

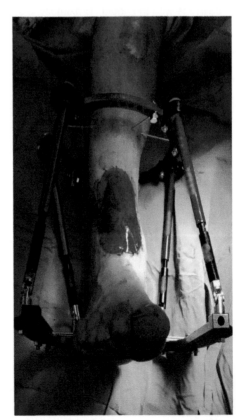

Fig. 17. Bilayer skin substitute applied to the anterior wound defect and immobilized with a static external fixator.

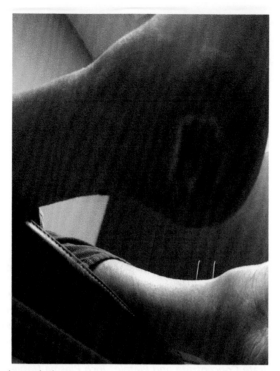

Fig. 18. Plantar calcaneal ulcer.

- Again, check with intraoperative Doppler to make sure the most distal perforator is still viable and has not been kinked during the flap rotation.
- The skin incision is closed primarily in layers. A closed suction drain can be used if intraoperative bleeding was not controlled adequately. Bilayer Wound Matrix (Integra) is placed on top of the muscle flap and secured with nonabsorbable sutures, and NPWT is applied on top of the Bilayer Wound Matrix at 125 mm Hg continuous suction (**Fig. 4**).

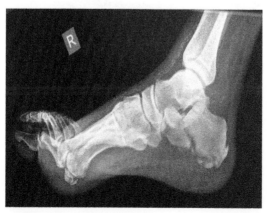

Fig. 19. Pathologic calcaneal fracture.

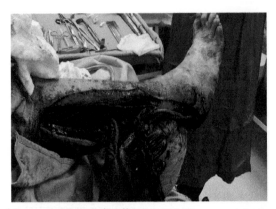

Fig. 20. Harvest of flap and rotating distally.

- A static circular external fixator is applied to the lower extremity for offloading, to limit movement at the muscle flap site and to allow for easy access during dressing changes (**Fig. 5**).
- The patient is placed on bed rest for at least 48 hours postoperatively, with gradual increase in dependency to help improve with venous return.
- If the recipient site remains viable in 10 days to 14 days postoperatively, the patient is brought back to the operating room for application of an STSG.

Bone Marrow Aspirate Concentrate and Platelet-Rich Plasma Harvest

- Intraoperatively, before inflation of the tourniquet (if the surgeon prefers using it for dissection when harvesting the PB muscle flap), approximately 30 mL to

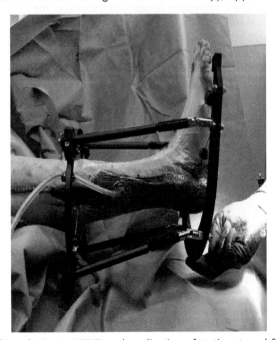

Fig. 21. Bilayer skin substitute, NPWT, and application of static external fixator.

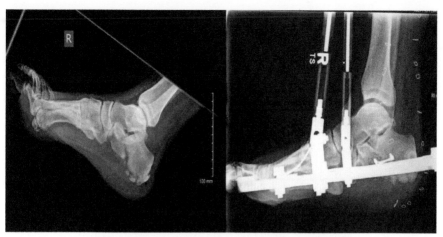

Fig. 22. Postoperative radiographs showing external fixator and ORIF of calcaneal fracture.

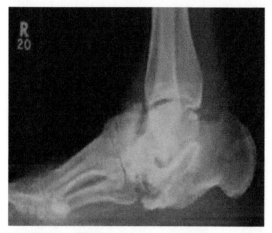

Fig. 23. Charcot ankle of 58-year-old man.

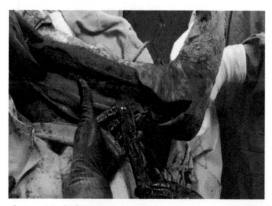

Fig. 24. Muscle flap harvest to help augment and increase vascularity to the arthrodesis site.

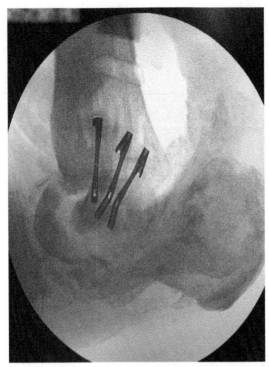

Fig. 25. Status post talectomy and compression staples for tibiocalcaneal fusion.

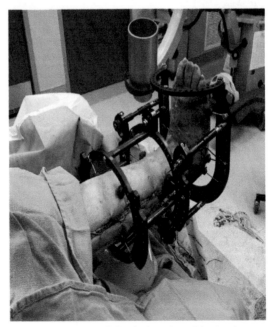

Fig. 26. Offloading and stabilization of the fusion site with circular external fixator.

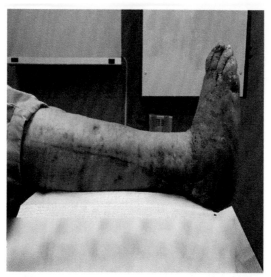

Fig. 27. Patient now has a braceable ankle and is ambulating in a CROW boot.

60 mL of bone marrow is obtained from the proximal medial tibial metaphysis, distal to the tibial tuberosity (**Fig. 6**).
- Using a Jamshidi needle, the tibial cortex is penetrated, and a syringe with approximately 2 mL of heparin is utilized to aspirate the bone marrow.
- The aspirated bone marrow is passed off the field and spun down per Magellan manufacturer specifications to yield between 3 mL and 10 mL of output volume of BMAC and PRP.

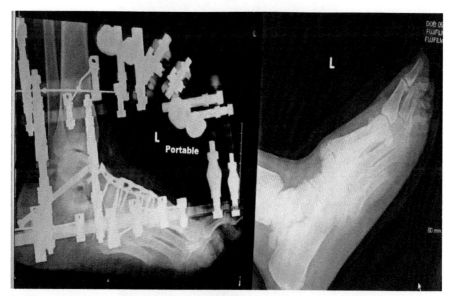

Fig. 28. .Charcot revision but failed 9 months later and now presents with an abscess.

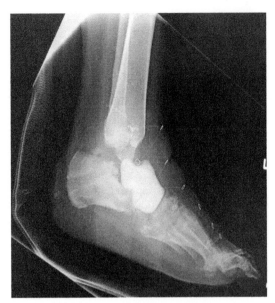

Fig. 29. Status post I&D with antibiotic-coated PMMA block.

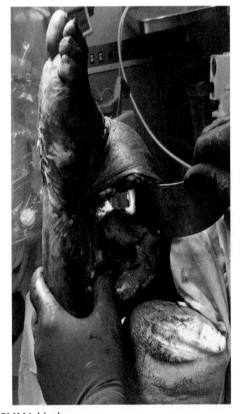

Fig. 30. Removal of PMMA block.

- The donor site wound bed and harvested muscle flap are infiltrated with the BMAC and PRP to augment healing (**Fig. 7**).

CLINICAL STUDIES
Case 1—Chronic Ulceration of Posterior Achilles Wound

A 62-year-old woman with a past medical history (PMH) of well-controlled type 2 diabetes mellitus (T2DM), osteoarthritis, and hypertension (HTN). The patient has had a right chronic posterior ulcer for approximately 2 years (**Fig. 8**). She has failed all local advanced wound care modalities and would like to pursue surgical intervention and limb salvage reconstruction. She had palpable pulses, and vascular studies revealed ankle-brachial index (ABI) of 0.92 to the right lower extremity. It was determined she would benefit from a staged PB muscle flap and STSG. The PB muscle flap was dissected and harvested as previously detailed, rotated distally, and tunneled subcutaneously to cover the posterior soft tissue defect (**Figs. 9** and **10**). Bilayer Wound Matrix and NPWT were utilized to augment healing. The surgical site is protected and immobilized with a static circular external fixator (**Figs. 11** and **12**). The patient was brought back approximately 4 weeks later for STSG harvest, application to the donor site with NPWT (**Fig. 13**). The patient's 2-year-old posterior Achilles wound was fully closed and healed in 14 weeks (**Fig. 14**).

Case 2—Chronic Anterior Ankle Ulceration

A 54-year-old man with a previous history of trimalleolar ankle open reduction and internal fixation (ORIF) suffered an anterior ankle wound dehiscence that remained open for approximately 1.5 years. The patient has a PMH of tobacco use and T2DM. He has failed all local advanced wound care modalities and would like to pursue surgical intervention and limb salvage reconstruction. He has palpable pulses and vascular studies revealed ABIs of 0.95 and good segmental pressures. He had multiple incisions and drainages (I&Ds) and all hardware from the ORIF was removed. The wound was converted to clean, with most recent culture showing no growth to date. Bone biopsies

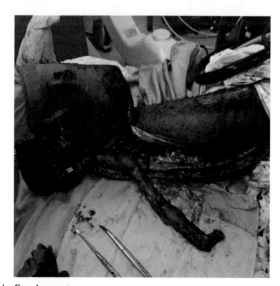

Fig. 31. PB muscle flap harvest.

were negative. It was determined that the patient would benefit from PB muscle flap and STSG. The PB muscle flap was dissected and harvested, as discussed previously, rotated distally, and tunneled subcutaneously to cover the anterior ankle soft tissue defect (**Figs. 15** and **16**). Bilayer Wound Matrix was utilized to augment and cover the muscle flap and then the surgical site protected and immobilized with a static circular external fixator (**Fig. 17**).

Case 3—Pathologic Calcaneal Fracture

A 64-year-old man with a plantar calcaneal ulcer for approximately 13 months presented to the clinic (**Fig. 18**). He has a PMH of T2DM, HTN, and coronary artery disease. Radiograph revealed that he has a pathologic calcaneal fracture (**Fig. 19**), probably due to OM. He has failed all local advanced wound care modalities and would like to pursue surgical intervention and limb salvage reconstruction. Patient has endovascular intervention with 2-vessel runoff to the foot, with 1 of them the peroneal artery. The wound was serially débrided until cultures were negative for any growth. Bone biopsies were positive for OM. It was determined patient would benefit from ORIF of the calcaneal fracture augmented with a PB muscle flap to treat the underlying chronic OM via vascularized delivery of intravenous antibiotics and offloading with external fixation. Bilayer Wound Matrix and NPWT then were utilized to accelerate the healing (**Figs. 20–22**). The patient went on to heal uneventfully, with the most recent bone biopsies negative for OM, in approximately 16 weeks.

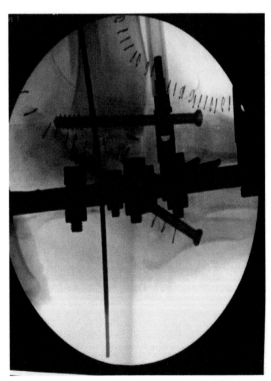

Fig. 32. Beaming lateral and medial column with 7.3-mm screws.

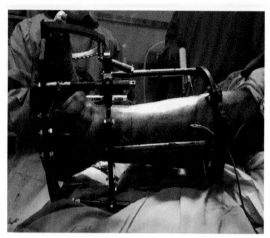

Fig. 33. All incision sites are closed up with application of a static external fixator.

Case 4—Peroneus Brevis Flap for Tibiocalcaneal Arthrodesis

A 58-year-old man with PMH of T2DM and Charcot foot on the right is referred for limb salvage Charcot reconstruction versus below-knee amputation. The patient has a 4-year history of Charcot breakdown regarding multiple I&Ds and offloading with a Charcot restraint orthotic walker (CROW) (**Fig. 23**). He currently has no open wounds. Pulses are palpable and vascular studies revealed ABIs of 0.82. A vascular consult was obtained, but no intervention is needed from a vascular standpoint, and patient is cleared for Charcot reconstruction. Bone biopsies were negative for OM but did show avascular necrosis of the talus. It then was determined that the patient would require a talectomy and tibiocalcaneal fusion, augmented with a PB muscle flap to increase vascularity to the fusion site, and offloading with a static circular external fixator

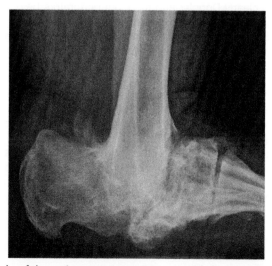

Fig. 34. Radiographs of the patient status post 2.5 years with functional and braceable limb.

(**Figs. 24–26**). The patient healed in 15 weeks and now has a braceable ankle and ambulates in a CROW (**Fig. 27**).

Case 5—Failed Charcot Revision

A 57-year-old man presented with a PMH of T2DM, Charcot foot, and OM. He had undergone a Charcot reconstruction approximately 9 months previously but now presents to clinic with a big abscess that required urgent I&D, talectomy, and application of antibiotic-coated polymethyl methacrylate (PMMA) block (**Figs. 28 and 29**). The patient underwent multiple débridements until culture results and bone biopsies were negative. He was brought back approximately 6 weeks later for staged PMMA antibiotic-coated bead removal and combined tibiocalcaneal and midfoot arthrodesis with a complementary PB muscle flap and external fixation (**Figs. 30–33**). The patient is now status post 2.5 years out with a functional and braceable limb (**Fig. 34**).

SUMMARY

The distally based PB muscle flap, as first described by Eren and colleagues[26] in 2001, has now widely been shown to be technically simple and reliable and has a fairly high success rate while minimizing donor site morbidity. It is an excellent alternative to fasciocutaneous, adipofascial, or free flaps in covering soft tissue defects in the lower extremity. Being a muscle flap, it is more versatile than the other flap options, discussed previously, due to having properties of conforming to the 3-dimensional defect, obliterating dead spaces, and improving host immunologic response by increasing local vascularity and antibiotic delivery. As with any flaps used in the lower extremity, the inherent risks, complications, and success rates are patient-dependent due to medical comorbidities, compliance, age, active local infection, and surgeon competency. In the correct hands, this flap can be a useful alternative in terms of limb salvage procedures versus amputation.

CLINICS CARE POINTS

- Make sure to clearly Doppler and mark out perforators before making the skin incision. This helps know the arc of rotation.
- The PB muscle flap is a versatile tool for diabetic limb salvage because it can help to cover large defects in the lower extremity.
- The distally based PB muscle flap has minimal morbidity and functional loss to the patient.
- Medical comorbidities, such as peripheral arterial disease, renal disease, diabetes mellitus, and smoking, can be detrimental to successful PB flap surgery and increase rate of failure. Therefore, patient selection is important to increase success rates and flap survivability.
- Other important parameters to take into considerations are the age of the patient, arc of rotation, surgical skills of the surgeon, tunneling of the flap, and inadequate preparation.
- Superficial necrosis of the flap is a common occurrence but can be treated easily with local wound care and débridement.

DISCLOSURE

The authors have nothing to disclose.

REFERENCES

1. Rodriguez Collazo ER, Bibbo C, Mechell RJ, et al. The reverse peroneus brevis muscle flap for ankle wound coverage. J Foot Ankle Surg 2013;52(4):543–6.
2. Nguyen T, Rodriguez-Collazo ER. Healing heel ulcers in high-risk patients: distally based peroneus brevis muscle flap case series. J Foot Ankle Surg 2019;58(2):341–6.
3. Lorenzetti F, Lazzeri D, Bonini L, et al. Distally based peroneus brevis muscle flap in reconstructive surgery of the lower leg: postoperative ankle function and stability evaluation. J Plast Reconstr Aesthet Surg 2010;63(9):1523–33.
4. Edgardo RRC, Jeffrey W, Tyler SM, et al. Peroneus brevis muscle flap with the use of INTEGRA® wound matrix and split thickness skin graft in the treatment of full thickness ulcerations: case reports and technique guide. Ortho Rheum Open Access J 2015;1(4):555567.
5. Clougherty C, et al. The Use of orthoplastic techniques for the treatment of lower extremity osteomyelitis and its response to inflammatory markers employing transitional muscle flaps. J Orthop Trauma Surg Relat Res 2018;13(1).
6. Ensat F, Hladik M, Larcher L, et al. The distally based peroneus brevis muscle flap—clinical series and review of the literature. Microsurgery 2014;34(3):203–8.
7. Schmidt AB, Giessler GA. The muscular and the new osteomuscular composite peroneus brevis flap: experiences from 109 cases. Plast Reconstr Surg 2010; 126(3):924–32.
8. Yang YL, Lin TM, Lee SS, et al. The distally pedicled peroneus brevis muscle flap anatomic studies and clinical applications. J Foot Ankle Surg 2005;44(4):259–64.
9. Ovaska MT, Madanat R, Tukiainen E, et al. Flap reconstruction for soft-tissue defects with exposed hardware following deep infection after internal fixation of ankle fractures. Injury 2014;45(12):2029–34.
10. Mukherjee MK, Parwaz MA, Chakravarty B, et al. Perforator flap: a novel method for providing skin coverage to lower limb defects. Med J Armed Forces India 2012;68:328–34.
11. Masadeh S, Christopher B. Distally based peroneus brevis flap: a reliable and versatile flap to cover the lateral foot and ankle. Curr Orthop Pract 2016;27(5): 499–507.
12. Rodriguez-Collazo E, et al. A systematic review of outcomes and flap selection following lower extremity free tissue transfer versus vascularized perforator pedicle flap transfer in lower limb reconstruction. Int J Orthop Surg 2018;1(2): 55–66.
13. Lai CS, Lin SD, Chou CK. Clinical application of the adipofascial turnover flap in the leg and ankle. Ann Plast Surg 1992;29:70–5.
14. Lin SD, Lai CS, Chiu YT, et al. Adipofascial flap of the lower leg based on the saphenous artery. Br J Plast Surg 1996;49:390–5.
15. Kim MB, Lee YH, Choi HS, et al. Distally-based medial crural adipofascial flap for coverage of medial foot and ankle. Arch Reconstr Microsurg 2015;24(2):56–61.
16. Sarhadi NS, Quaba AA. Experience with the adipofascial turn-over flap. Br J Plast Surg 1993;46:307–13.
17. Klebuc M, Menn Z. Muscle flaps and their role in limb salvage. Methodist Debakey Cardiovasc J 2013;9(2):95.
18. ElGhamry AH. Peroneal tendofascial flap: a new fascial flap for Achilles tendon coverage, a preliminary report. Br J Plast Surg 2003;56(3):284–8.
19. Hu XH, Du WL, Chen Z, et al. The application of distally pedicled peroneus brevis muscle flaps and retrograde neurocutaneous accompanying artery flaps for

treatment of bony and soft-tissue 3-dimensional defects of the lower leg and foot. Int J Low Extrem Wounds 2013;12(1):53–62.

20. Thordarson DB, Patzakis MJ, Holtom P, et al. Salvage of the septic ankle with concomitant tibial osteomyelitis. Foot Ankle Int 1997;18(3):151–6.

21. Mathes SJ, Alpert BS, Chang N. Use of the muscle flap in chronic osteomyelitis: experimental and clinical correlation. Plast Reconstr Surg 1982;69(5):815–28.

22. Ng YH, Chong KW, Tan GM, et al. Distally pedicled peroneus brevis muscle flap: a versatile lower leg and foot flap. Singapore Med J 2010;51(4):339.

23. Wagner T, Hupkens P, Slater NJ, et al. The proximally based long peroneal muscle turnover flap: a novel salvage flap for small to medium-sized defects of the knee. J Plast Reconstr Aesthet Surg 2016;69:533–7.

24. Bach AD, Leffler M, Kneser U, et al. The versatility of the distally based peroneus brevis muscle flap in reconstructive surgery of the foot and lower leg. Ann Plast Surg 2007;58(4):397–404.

25. Mathes SJ, Nahai F. Classification of the vascular anatomy of muscles: experimental and clinical correlation. Plast Reconstr Surg 1981;67:177–87.

26. Eren S, Ghofrani A, Reifenrath M. The distally pedicled peroneus brevis muscle flap: a new flap for the lower leg. Plast Reconstr Surg 2001;107:1443–8.

27. Koski EA, Kuokkanen HO, Tukiainen EJ. Distally-based peroneus brevis muscle flap: a successful way of reconstructing lateral soft tissue defects of the ankle. Scand J Plast Reconstr Surg Hand Surg 2005;39:299e301.

28. Taylor GI, Pan WR. Angiosomes of the leg: anatomic study and clinical implications. Plast Reconstr Surg 1998;102:599–616.

29. Gosau M, Schoeneich M, Koyama K, et al. Ultrasound analyses, anatomical considerations, and clinical experience with theperoneus brevis muscle flap. Ann Anat 2013;195(2):183–8.

The Distally Based Posterior Tibial Artery Flap

William C. Perry, DPM[a],*, Suhail Masadeh, DPM[a], Alessandro Thione, MD, PhD[b]

KEYWORDS

- Medial leg fasciocutaneous flap • Posterior tibial artery • Lower limb reconstruction
- Limb salvage • Perforator

KEY POINTS

- Inclusion of the great saphenous vein and saphenous nerve improves perfusion to flap and allows further advancement.
- Management of postoperative venous congestion is key to survival of these flaps.
- Anesthesia overlying the saphenous nerve distribution of the anterior medial ankle and dorsal medial foot is to be expected.
- Multiple posterior tibial artery perforators can be found 5 to 10 cm proximal to the medial malleolus.
- Maintain distance from most proximal perforator and pivot point of at least 2 cm to prevent compression/kinking of the perforators with a turndown flap.

INTRODUCTION

Soft tissue defects of the lower leg and hindfoot are challenging due to superficial tendon, bone, and neurovascular structures. The use of fasciocutaneous flaps for coverage of distal leg/hindfoot tissue defects has numerous advantages over alternative options muscle or free flaps. As compared with muscle flaps, the fasciocutaneous flaps result in no loss of function, provides higher patient satisfaction and aesthetic result,[1] and has a significantly faster return to weight bearing.[2] In contrast to free flaps, coverage of the distal leg with perforator flaps allows a shorter hospital stay postoperatively,[3] requires less operative time inherently reducing costs, and carries less risk for perioperative cardiac and pulmonary complications.[4]

Distally based fasciocutaneous flaps of the leg have been described in the literature, with the most common being the peroneal propeller flap and the reverse sural artery flap. However, the medial fasciocutaneous flaps of the leg based on perfusion of the

[a] Cincinnati Veteran Affairs Medical Center, 3200 Vine Street, Cincinnati, OH 45220, USA;
[b] Department of Plastic Surgery and Burns, Hospital Universitari i Politecnic La Fe, 106 Avinguda de Fernando Abril Martorell, Valencia E-46026, Spain
* Corresponding author.
E-mail address: William.perry24a467@va.gov

Clin Podiatr Med Surg 37 (2020) 671–680
https://doi.org/10.1016/j.cpm.2020.05.003
0891-8422/20/Published by Elsevier Inc.

posterior tibial artery are gaining popularity as the simplest, most robust flap available for the coverage of traumatic wounds, oncologic resections, and exposed orthopedic hardware to the distal leg.[5,6]

The posterior tibial artery flap was first described by Zhang[7] in 1983. This initial design used a fasciocutaneous flap elevated as a free flap along with the arterial trunk of the posterior tibial artery. Although the flap was considered a success, sacrificing an important primary vessel in the lower extremity limited its use due to significant donor site risks. In the early 1990s Koshima and Soeda, and later Masquelet, described the use of posterior tibial artery perforators that could support a large flap without compromising major vessels.[8,9] Since this description, the medial fasciocutaneous perforator flaps of the leg have been used as a free flap,[10] cross-leg flaps,[11] island propeller flaps,[6] and turndown adipofascial flaps,[12] all with good results. The posterior tibial perforator flap has gained popularity for soft tissue defects in the lower leg and some consider it to be the preferred fasciocutaneous flap.[5,6]

The medial leg offers a broad area for harvest of a fasciocutaneous flap with adequate reach tissues for coverage of the inferior heel, achilles tendon, medial and anterior ankle, and dorsal midfoot wounds. The distally based posterior tibial artery perforator flap is perfused by septocutaneous perforators that supply adjacent deep fascia, adipose, and cutaneous tissues to the medial and posterior leg.[8,13,14]

ANATOMY OF THE POSTERIOR TIBIAL FASCIOCUTANEOUS FLAP

The posterior tibial artery is one of the terminating branches of the popliteal artery originating distal to the popliteal fossa. It travels within the deep posterior compartment of the leg and terminates just distal to the tarsal tunnel before branching into the plantar pedal arteries. In the deep posterior compartment the posterior tibial artery lies between the flexor digitorum longus and soleus muscles, sending perforators to the overlying medial-posterior leg. These posterior tibial artery perforators can be direct cutaneous, septocutaneous, or musculocutaneous.[15] The posterior tibial artery angiosome has the largest number of perforating arteries to the middle and distal leg as compared with the peroneal and anterior tibial artery angiosomes.[16] The 2 larger distal septocutaneous perforators of the posterior tibial artery are located in the range of 4 to 8 cm superior to the medial malleolus,[17] allowing good perfusion to a distally based flap and can be readily dopplerable.

A single perforator supplies a perforasome via the subdermal plexus. It is within the adipose and fascial network that the microvascular network allows an area of tissue perfusion without the requirement of a major axial vessel. Perforators of the posterior tibial artery are usually found in 3 distinct clusters in the leg: 4 to 9 cm, 13 to 18 cm, and 21 to 26 cm from the intermalleolar line. Each section contains at least 23% of the total number of perforators.[13] The deep fascia component of the flap carries a microvascular network that is able to sustain a much longer flap as opposed to a cutaneous flap and can be elevated with a subcutaneous adipose layer to maintain a thick durable flap.[18–21]

When large defects to the distal leg or foot require coverage, surgeons have incorporated an axial vascular network based on the saphenous nerve to extend the length and size of the medial leg fasciocutaneous flap.[22–24] Within this same perforasome of the posterior tibial perforators is an axial vascular network running longitudinal with the leg, supplied by the great saphenous vein and saphenous nerve. The saphenous nerve and vein have axial nutrient arteries known as "vasa vasorum" and "vasa nervorum."

These arterial networks are supplied by 11 unique sources via deep fascia, periosteum, and cutaneous branches and are supplied by the posterior tibial artery and the branches of the descending genicular artery.[7,25] Inclusion of this perineural vascular network improves circulation of the flap.

CLINICAL APPLICATION AND SURGICAL TECHNIQUE

Using an 8MHZ acoustic doppler preoperatively, distal perforators of the posterior tibial artery can be readily identified. For a turndown or propeller based flap of the distal leg, perforators that are 5 to 10 cm proximal to the malleolar line must be patent and outside of the zone of injury/defect. Marking these perforators can be done preoperatively using a skin marker. For large turndown, or turnover flaps, there is no need for microsurgery, and the direct identification of these perforators intraoperatively is not beneficial. Color dopplers, computed tomography angiography, and angiograms provide additional information as to the overall perfusion of the distal extremity if concerns for peripheral vascular disease exist secondary to atherosclerosis or history of trauma.

An approximate pivot point should be measured for a distally based turndown flap, with a minimum of 2 cm margin proximal to the perforator to minimize vascular kinking with transposition.[23] An additional 1 to 2 cm should be added to the overall length of the flap to allow good coverage of the defect and allow approximation without tension once transposed.

These flaps are usually performed under general anesthesia or spinal anesthesia to allow for a thigh tourniquet. Depending on the tissue defect, the position of the patient can be supine or prone. Stabilization of osseous structures should be performed before flap elevation. If transposing the flap across a primary axis of a joint, such as the ankle, immobilization with external fixation is recommended.

A linear incision is made along the course of the medial leg posterior to the great saphenous vein and anterior to the posterior tibial artery perforators that are approximately 2 to 3 cm posterior to the vein. The authors prefer to use this flap as an adipofascial flap to allow primary closure of the donor site and to stage the flap for a split-thickness skin graft. Skin edges are elevated with a 2-mm adipose layer to prevent delamination of the skin at the donor site. The adipofascial flap can be incised starting proximally with ligation of the great saphenous vein and saphenous nerve developed medial and laterally. In order to avoid exposure of the medial face of the tibia or damage to the underlying periosteum, the authors suggest maintaining a minimum 1.5 cm distance from the tibial crest.

The flap is then elevated with the deep fascia. Dissection is carried distally to the pivot point with care taken to preserve at least 1 to 2 perforators distal perforators. The flap is turned down and inset into the defect for approximation of defect coverage. The great saphenous vein is preserved if the flap is thick enough but it is included and ligated at the base of the flap if it is thin to avoid venous congestion.[5] The authors do not recommend tunneling under a skin bridge, as postoperative venous congestion to the leg and flap can lead to flap necrosis. The width of the pedicle should be wide enough to allow perfusion through subcutaneous tissues and fascia and perineural vascular network. The flap base/length ratio of 3:1 is the traditional approach, and ratios up to 4:1 are frequently successful.[24] The consensus for pedicle width for large distally based flaps is a minimum of 3 to 4 cm.[11,26,27]

Before transposition, the tourniquet is lowered, and if vasospasm occurs with absence of dopplerable pulse, the flap should be given 10 minutes to recover.

The use of vasodilators such as lidocaine, papaverine, nitro paste, or warm saline placed around the pedicle to alleviate a vasospasm as well as to promote the dilation of additional vascular channels within the flap is recommended. If vasospasm persists, the flap is returned to the harvest site and delayed for later transposition.

In addition, the management of postoperative venous congestion of the flap is imperative to prevent necrosis. Numerous approaches to the effective management of this occurrence are described in the literature, including postoperative phlebotomy, leech therapy, negative pressure wound therapy, valvotomy, vein supercharging, and ligation of proximal and distal ends of the axial vein with good success. Resulting partial necrosis to flap margins is usually managed with local wound care and delayed split-thickness skin grafting.[11,22] It is believed that it is imperative to adhere to the saphenous vein dissection described earlier in order to effectively avoid venous congestion.

Residual anesthesia is to be expected in the distal leg after sectioning of the saphenous nerve within the flap. Depending on the defect location the saphenous nerve included in the reverse flap can be coapted with a sural nerve in heel defect coverage for ensuring the protective sensation of the zone of injury to make a sensate flap.[11] Inclusion of the perineural vascular network, while sparing the saphenous nerve, has been described; however, this requires extensive dissection.

CASE STUDY #1

A 26-year-old man was injured in a motor vehicle accident in a third-world country. The injury resulted in extensive degloving of the midfoot and hindfoot with loss of the fourth and fifth rays (**Fig. 1**). Initial debridement consisted of the amputation of the fourth and fifth metatarsals, followed by local wound care. Because of the absence of necessary surgeons in that country to provide a definitive procedure, local wound care was continued for 4 months. As part of a medical missions program, this patient was selected for reconstruction due to concerns of limb loss, given his nonviable

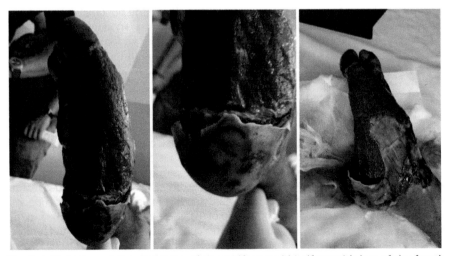

Fig. 1. Initial injury of the degloving of the midfoot and hindfoot with loss of the fourth and fifth rays.

plantar heel pad. The distally based posterior tibial artery flap was chosen for primary coverage of the heel after a thorough doppler examination was performed. The flap was incised and elevated as a turndown fasciocutaneous flap including the great saphenous vein and saphenous nerve within the flap (**Fig. 2**). This flap was then transposed and inset to the inferior heel. Split-thickness skin grafts were used for the plantar arch and dorsal foot, and the donor site of the posterior tibial artery flap was closed primarily. No flap loss or necrosis was evident, and postoperative venous congestion to the flap was resolved with intermittent phlebotomy in the first 48 hours. The patient healed uneventfully with a viable flap and skin grafts (**Fig. 3**).

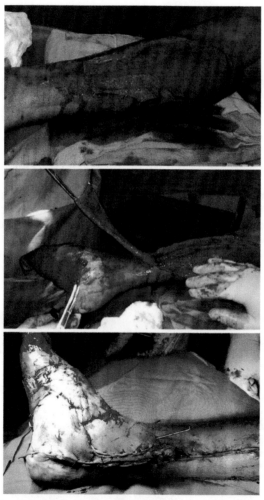

Fig. 2. Turndown fasciocutaneous flap including the great saphenous vein and saphenous nerve.

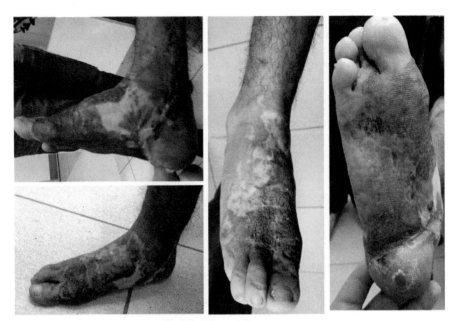

Fig. 3. Healed fasciocutaneous flap and skin grafts.

CASE STUDY #2

A 50-year-old diabetic man with a history of a Lisfranc amputation developed a decubitus heel ulcer (**Fig. 4**). Following excisional wound debridement, a posterior tibial artery perforator flap was elevated and transposed with a small cutaneous paddle. The adjacent pedicle was covered loosely with an integra bilayer graft. During the postoperative period, venous congestion of the flap led to partial necrosis of the cutaneous paddle, which was debrided and covered using a delayed split-thickness skin graft (**Fig. 5**).

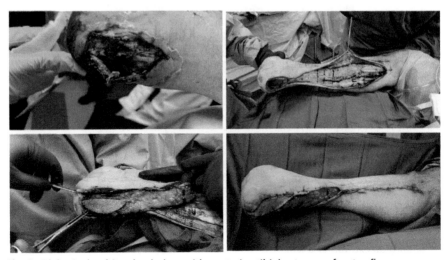

Fig. 4. Diabetic decubitus heel ulcer with posterior tibial artery perforator flap.

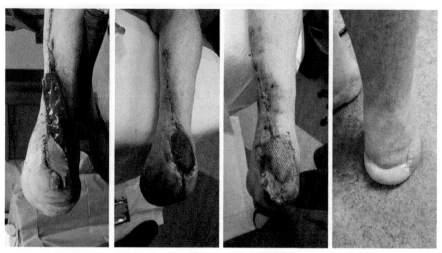

Fig. 5. A delayed split-thickness skin graft covering partial necrosis of the cutaneous paddle.

CASE STUDY #3

A patient with a large leiomyosarcoma proximal to the anterior ankle presented with a subcutaneous mass, approximately 5 cm in diameter. The mass was noted to be firm, mobile, nontender, and nontranslucent without dilated veins. Surgical excision was performed (**Fig. 6**), frozen sections were sent for evaluation, and clear margins were obtained. Immediate intraoperative coverage of the soft tissue defect was performed using the posterior tibial artery perforator flap and skin graft. Postoperatively, ankle range of motion was maintained and the flap healed without complication.

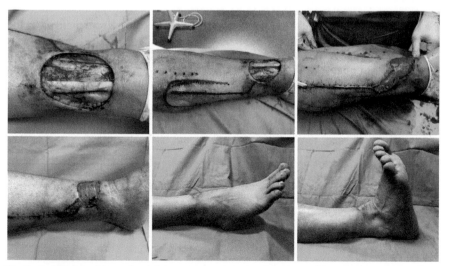

Fig. 6. Surgical excision of a leiomyosarcoma to the anterior ankle, maintaining range of motion.

DISCUSSION

Soft tissue defects to the distal leg and hindfoot are challenging with only the smallest defects closed primarily without tissue transposition. These defects to the distal leg and hindfoot can lead to tendon desiccation, damaged neurovascular structures, and exposed joint surfaces. These wounds can also be the result of postoperative dehiscence and exposed orthopedic hardware, making it susceptible to infection. Expeditious primary coverage of these defects will allow return to function and avoid limb loss. Pedicled fasciocutaneous flaps of the medial leg provide an excellent solution with good outcomes that do not require microanastomosis and have similar outcomes as compared with free flap reconstruction in the lower extremity.[28] The medial leg provides tissue transfer with multiple perforators of the posterior tibial artery and axial perineural vascular networks allowing coverage of large defect areas with greater arc of rotation.[10]

The evolution of the posterior tibial artery flap, to include the saphenous vein and nerve and its suprafascial axial vascular network, allows further transposition and increased flap dimensions. The saphenous neurovascular bundle is a robust vascular plexus supplied by 11 distinct arterial sources.[7] By including this axial supply, in combination with the posterior tibial artery distal perforators, a length to width ratio of 4:1 has been shown to have reliable success in increasing the size of the fasciocutaneous flap for the distal leg.[24]

The dissection, elevation, and transposition of the posterior tibial adipofascial flap can be performed with relative ease and, with the inclusion of the perineural vascular network, constitutes a robust flap for coverage of large defects in the distal leg and hindfoot.

CLINICAL CARE POINTS

- Inclusion of the great saphenous vein and saphenous nerve improves perfusion to flap and allows further advancement.
- Management of postoperative venous congestion is key to survival of these flaps.
- Anesthesia overlying the saphenous nerve distribution of the anterior medial ankle and dorsal medial foot is to be expected.
- Multiple posterior tibial artery perforators can be found 5 to 10 cm proximal to the medial malleolus.
- Maintain distance from most proximal perforator and pivot point of at least 2 cm to prevent compression/kinking of the perforators with a turndown flap.

DISCLOSURE

The authors have nothing to disclose.

REFERENCE

1. Buono P, Castus P, Dubois-Ferrière V. Muscular versus non-muscular free flaps for soft tissue coverage of chronic tibial osteomyelitis. World J Plast Surg 2018; 7(3):294–300.

2. Paro J, Chiou G, Subhro S. Comparing muscle and fasciocutaneous free flaps in lower extremity reconstruction—does it matter? Ann Plast Surg 2016;76:S213–5.

3. Bhatti A, Adeshola A, Ismael T, et al. Lower leg flaps comparison between free versus local flaps. Internet J Plast Surg 2006;3(2):1–8.

4. Parrett BM, Winograd JM, Lin SJ, et al. The posterior tibial artery perforator flap: an alternative to free-flap closure in the comorbid patient. J Reconstr Microsurg 2009;25(02):105–9.

5. Cavadas PC. Reversed saphenous neurocutaneous island flap: clinical experience and evolution to the posterior tibial perforator-saphenous subcutaneous flap. Plast Reconstr Surg 2003;111(2):837–9.

6. Robotti E, Carminati M, Bonfirraro PP, et al. "On demand" posterior tibial artery perforator flaps: a versatile surgical procedure for reconstruction of soft tissue defects of the leg after tumor excision. Ann Plast Surg 2010;64(2):202–9.

7. Zhang SC. Clinical application of medial skin flap of leg–analysis of 9 cases. Zhonghua Wai Ke Za Zh 1983;21(12):743–5.

8. Koshima I, Moriguchi T, Ohta S. The vasculature and clinical application of the posterior tibial perforator-based flap. J Plast Reconstr Surg 1992;90(4):643–9.

9. Masquelet AC, Romana MC, Wolf G. Skin island flaps supplied by the vascular axis of the sensitive superficial nerves: anatomic study and clinical experience in the leg. Plast Reconstr Surg 1993;89(6):1115–21.

10. Hung LK, Lao J, Ho PC. Free posterior tibial perforator flap: anatomy and a report of 6 cases. Microsurgery 1996;17(9):503–11.

11. Goil P, Choudhary GM, Jain R, et al. Versatile distally based neurocutaneous saphenous flap in the era of microsurgery. Eur J Plast Surg 2018;41(2):165–72.

12. Lu S, Wang C, Wen G, et al. Versatility of the greater saphenous fasciocutaneous perforator flap in coverage of the lower leg. J Reconstr Microsurg 2014;30(03):179–86.

13. Schaverien M, Saint-Cyr M. Perforators of the lower leg: analysis of perforator locations and clinical application for pedicled perforator flaps. Plast Reconstr Surg 2008;122(1):161–70.

14. Parrett BM, Winograd JM, Lin SJ, et al. A review of local and regional flaps for distal leg reconstruction. J Reconstr Microsurg 2009;25(7):445–55.

15. Yousif NJ, Ye Z. Analysis of cutaneous perfusion: an aid to lower extremity reconstruction. Clin Plast Surg 1991;18:559.

16. Tapadar A, Palit S, Kundu R, et al. A study of the perforating arteries of the leg derived from the anterior tibial, posterior tibial and peroneal arteries. J Anat Soc India 2014;63(1):43–7.

17. Niranjan NS. Posterior tibial artery perforator flap. In: Wei FC, Mardini S, editors. Flaps and reconstructive surgery. 2nd edition. Edinburgh (Scotland): Elsevier; 2017. p. 717–28.

18. Pontén B. The fasciocutaneous flap: its use in soft tissue defects of the lower leg. Br J Plast Surg 1981;34(2):215–20.

19. Barclay T, Cardoso E, Sharpe D, et al. Repair of lower leg injuries with fasciocutaneous flaps. Br J Plast Surg 1982;35(2):127–32.

20. Thatte RL, Laud N. The use of the fascia of the lower leg as a roll-over flap. Plast Reconstr Surg 1985;75(3):455.

21. Lai CS, Lin SD, Yang CC, et al. Adipofascial turn-over flap for reconstruction of the dorsum of the foot. Br J Plast Surg 1991;44(3):170–4.

22. Kansal S, Goil P, Agarwal V, et al. Reverse pedicle-based greater saphenous neuro-veno-fasciocutaneous flap for reconstruction of lower leg and foot. Eur J Orthop Surg Traumatol 2014;24(1):67–72.

23. Zhong W, Lu S, Wang C, et al. Single perforator greater saphenous neuro-veno-fasciocutaneous propeller flaps for lower extremity reconstructions. ANZ J Surg 2017;87(7- 8):E40–5.

24. Foo TL, Chew WYC, Tan BK. Improving the reliability of the distally based posterior tibial artery adipofascial flap with the great saphenous venoneural network. Ann Plast Surg 2011;67(3):288–93.

25. Huang WC, Chen HC, Wei FC, et al. Chimeric flap in clinical use. Clin Plast Surg 2003;30(3):457–67.

26. Shao X, Yu Y, Zhang X, et al. Repair of soft-tissue defect close to the distal perforating artery using the modified distally based medial fasciocutaneous flap in the distal lower leg. J Reconstr Microsurg 2011;27(03):145–50.

27. Dai J, Chai Y, Wang C, et al. Comparative study of two types of distally based sural neurocutaneous flap for reconstruction of lower leg, ankle, and heel. J Reconstr Microsurg 2013;29(02):125–30.

28. Nenad T, Reiner W, Michael S, et al. Saphenous perforator flap for reconstructive surgery in the lower leg and the foot: a clinical study of 50 patients with posttraumatic osteomyelitis. J Trauma 2010;68(5):1200–7.

Peroneal Artery Adipofascial Flaps for Coverage of Distal Leg and Rearfoot

Ramy X. Fahim, DPM[a,b,]*, Sharif R. AbdelFattah, DPM[c,d]

KEYWORDS

- Adipofascial • Flap • Peroneal • Tibial • Wound • Wound care • Free flap

KEY POINTS

- Peroneal artery adipofascial flaps are useful alternatives for coverage of small to moderately sized defects of the lower extremity.
- Adipofascial flaps can be a reliable and effective way to provide early closure of a wound, preventing chronic wound healing issues and potentially limb-threatening osteomyelitis.
- The benefits of use of adipofascial flaps rather than muscle flaps is that there is no resultant loss of function and significantly faster return to weight bearing.
- Compared with free flaps, adipofascial flaps have similar failure and complication rates.
- The combination of ease of technique, limited donor site morbidity, and more cosmetically appealing outcome results in a more satisfactory outcome for the patient.

PERONEAL ARTERY ADIPOFASCIAL FLAPS FOR COVERAGE OF DISTAL LEG AND HINDFOOT

Chronic and difficult-to-heal wounds of the lower extremity pose several challenges for practitioners interested in limb salvage. These presenting defects can be confounded by exposed muscle, tendon, bone, or hardware or a combination enhancing the difficulty and potential for complication. In addition, the attempts at wound healing are often compounded by infection, sensory neuropathy, and local ischemia, which, in order to resolve, requires a more multifaceted approach. Many times, these defects are either directly or indirectly the result of complicating patient factors that impair the wound's healing potential. These patients have often failed multiple conservative modalities of therapy, been deemed inappropriate candidates for primary closure, failed use of negative pressure wound therapy, or experienced failure

[a] Foot and Ankle Surgery, Mercy Health, Youngstown, OH, USA; [b] Northern Ohio Medical Specialties (NOMS) Healthcare, Sandusky, OH, USA; [c] East Liverpool City Hospital, East Liverpool, OH, USA; [d] Sullivan County Community Hospital, 2200 North Section Street, Sullivan, IN 47882, USA
* Corresponding author. 1700 East Market Street, Warren, OH 44483.
E-mail address: RFahim0181@gmail.com

Clin Podiatr Med Surg 37 (2020) 681–697
https://doi.org/10.1016/j.cpm.2020.07.005
podiatric.theclinics.com

with the use of dermal matrices. In these cases, these patients necessitate consideration of more robust and definitive methods of wound closure. Often, the question of amputation may be posed by the practitioner; however, there are techniques that may be used at lower risk to the patient and that potentially avoid a life-altering amputation.[1]

According to the reconstructive triangle proposed by Mathes and Nahai[2] and the reconstructive elevator introduced by Gottlieb and Kreiger,[3] there is a systematic approach that should be taken in order to enhance the possibility of wound closure. Wong and Niranjan[4] suggested that these rungs of the ladder and advancement of steps should not be sequential because of the varying degrees of the surgeon's skill set.[5] Soft tissue flaps are useful for several purposes in limb reconstruction and limb salvage. They allow perfusion to a site that may previously have been avascular, allowing delivery of host immunity factors and systemic antibiotics. In addition, they provide stability to a site of injury via host growth factors, osteogenic progenitors from muscular and adipose mesenchymal stem cells that are conducive to bone regeneration. The interposition of soft tissue between dead space or bony prominences further helps to protect the soft tissue and underlying structures from pressure injury.

A wide variety of local flaps have been described and used to reconstruct wounds of the lower extremity. Free tissue transfers could provide adequate coverage for these defects; however, these leave undesirable results at the donor site and require more

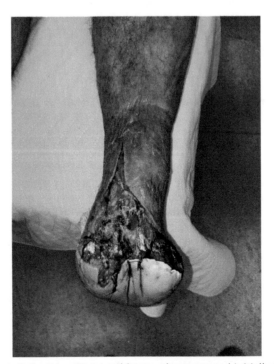

Fig. 1. Case study 1. Patient is a 61-year-old man who presented initially for gas gangrene extending to his proximal midfoot. Following initial decompression incision and drainage and guillotine amputation at the level of the Chopart joint, the patient was medically stabilized and a thorough vascular work-up was performed. The wound is shown before surgical intervention. (*Courtesy of* R. Fahim DPM, Warren, OH.)

technical skill.[6,7] In a meta-analysis, Bekara and colleagues[8] found similar failure and overall complication rates for perforator propeller flaps compared with free flaps. Transposition, advancement flaps, and rotational flaps are limited in their ability to cover large defects and limited range of mobilization.[9,10] Muscle flaps are another viable option in attempts to reconstruct the lower extremity; however, compared with fasciocutaneous or adipofascial flaps, a major downside is the loss of function that results from harvesting that muscle. Aesthetically, there is a downside to using muscle rather than fasciocutaneous or adipofascial flaps.[11] Fasciocutaneous flaps have significant donor site morbidity and require grafting of the donor site, leading to less aesthetic appeal.

The presence of multiple perforator alternatives around the distal leg has resulted in versatility in choice and selection of flaps. This versatility allows variability in size and location of defect reconstruction.[12] There is none of the disruption to the major vessels or musculature that is often required with a muscle or free flap. The distally based adipofascial flap is an excellent option for reconstruction. Cavadas and colleagues[13] proposed that the medially based adipofascial flap is the easiest and most versatile flap for coverage at the ankle. These flaps are thin and do not require microsurgical expertise, thus are easy to mobilize. In addition to ease of harvest, the donor site can be primarily closed at the initial time of harvest and mobilization, resulting in a superior cosmetic result.

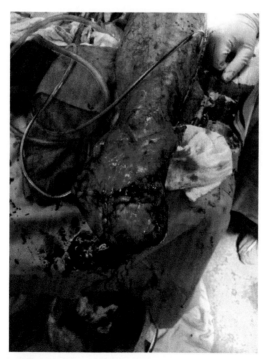

Fig. 2. Case study 1. Primary closure of the donor site from the lateral aspect of the leg following harvest of the adipofascial flap and placing a drain. The adipofascial flap shows its arc of rotation across the anterior distal tibia to cover the exposed bone at the distal medial aspect of the amputation site. (*Courtesy of* R. Fahim DPM, Warren, OH.)

Not only is it aesthetically desirable but the adipofascial flap is recognized for its reliability and durability. Schmidt and colleagues[14] found that adipofascial flaps are just as durable as fasciocutaneous flaps in non–weight-bearing and weight-bearing areas. Paro and colleagues[15] did a study comparing return to weight bearing with muscle flaps versus fasciocutaneous free flaps and found that there was a significantly expedited return to weight bearing with the fasciocutaneous group compared with muscle flaps. Adipofascial flaps are a reliable way of providing a vascularized bed for skin grafts when a patient is not a suitable candidate for muscle or free flap. In addition to stability and aesthetics, these flaps are useful because of the lack of significant bulk that prevents ease of using shoe gear and socks. Use of debulked adipofascial tissue for coverage has merit compared with other options such as fasciocutaneous flap, muscle, and myocutaneous flap in this regard.

The benefits of this adipofascial flap also are related to variability in harvesting technique. The ability to have a wide arc of rotation is advantageous and it does not always require a pivot point.[7,9,10,12] An alternative is using a turn-down or turn-over technique to transfer the flap, which helps to avoid kinking or skeletonization of the perforator. Beyond the sural flap, which is the most popular for lower extremity reconstruction, there are 2 other valuable flaps: the posterior tibial artery and peroneal artery perforator adipofascial flaps.

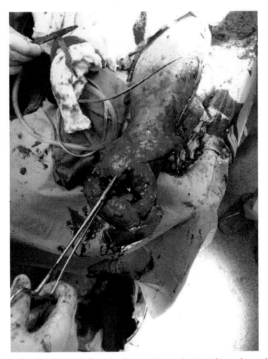

Fig. 3. Case study 1. The harvested flap is shown in order to show length and coverage of the medial aspect of the amputation site where there was exposed bone. The arc of rotation of the adipofascial flap can be seen for the lateral aspect of the leg to the distal anterior medial amputation site. (*Courtesy of* R. Fahim DPM, Warren, OH.)

PERONEAL ARTERY FASCIOCUTANEOUS FLAP FOR COVERAGE OF THE DISTAL LEG AND HINDFOOT

Chronic defects of the lateral aspect of the leg or hindfoot can be addressed using the peroneal artery adipofascial flap. The lateral aspect of the lower extremity can have several challenging presentations. Exposed tendon, bone, or metal fixation from fibular fractures that often fail to heal in an appropriate amount of time is one of the more common problematic presentations. In addition, there is a lack of soft tissue available for adequate coverage at and around the level of the ankle. The patient population with these chronic nonhealing wounds may have several medical and social issues that further complicate the healing process. Perfusion of the lower extremity is a significant consideration that, when impaired, contributes to poor wound healing capabilities. Yoshimura and colleagues[16] were the first to describe the peroneal artery perforator flap based on peroneal artery angiosomes. This flap helps to preserve muscle function, spares major vessels, has variability within its design, and has enhanced mobility compared with the other types of flaps that are available. Because microsurgical techniques are not used with adipofascial flaps, it tends to be less time consuming than other complex techniques. High vascularity of the flap has the added benefit of direct delivery of parenterally administered antibiotic in cases of osteomyelitis or exposed metal. Lin and colleagues[17] initially described the distally based

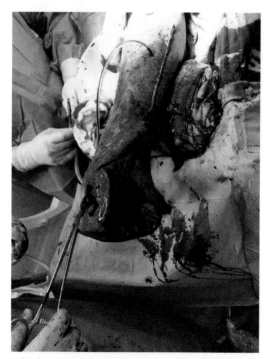

Fig. 4. Case study 1. The harvested flap is shown in order to show length and coverage of the medial aspect of the amputation site where there was exposed bone. The arc of rotation of the adipofascial flap can be seen for the lateral aspect of the leg to the distal anterior medial amputation site. (*Courtesy of* R. Fahim DPM, Warren, OH.)

adipofascial flap perforator of the peroneal artery with excellent results in short-term follow-up for small defects.

Another noted benefit of this flap, when the turn-down technique is used, is that it exposes the undersurface of the overturned flap to adipose tissue, which, in the case of exposed tendon, allows free mobilization without fear of adhesion, whereas the outer fascia can accept skin grafts readily.[9] Lee and colleagues[7] described their success using adipofascial turn-down flaps for use in larger defects with longer-term follow-up. Li and colleagues[18] showed that, for complicated wounds of the distal third of the lower leg, foot, and ankle region, these adipofascial turn-down flaps can be durable even in patients with multiple comorbidities, including diabetes mellitus, tobacco abuse, and osteomyelitis, with an average of 14-month follow-up.

Anatomic Considerations

Purushothaman and colleagues[19] investigated the anatomy of the peroneal artery perforators. They were able to show that there was some consistency in the way that septocutaneous perforators were distributed from the terminal aspect of the peroneal artery. The peroneal artery is one of the terminal branches of the tibiofibular trunk. The peroneal artery runs within the deep posterior compartment of the leg. Batchelor and Moss[20] were able to describe the subfascial plexus, intrafascial plexus, and perifascial plexus and their levels of perfusion. The peroneal artery flap is a type B adipofascial flap when harvested. It can measure 10 × 20 cm with a pedicle that is 3 cm long

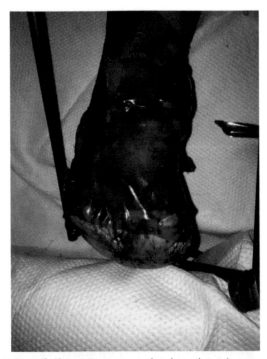

Fig. 5. Case study 1. Once the harvest was secured, a dermal matrix was used for coverage of the adipofascial flap in order to stimulate granulation tissue for the recipient skin graft to be planned in the near future. At this time, an external fixator was placed in order to stabilize the graft while the wound healed in order to prevent any shearing forces from the ankle joint range of motion that would result in failure. (Photo courtesy of Dr. Ramy Fahim.)

and has a diameter of 0.5 mm.[21] In the distally based lateral adipofascial flap, septocutaneous perforators of the peroneal artery are the primary source of perfusion. Batchelor and Moss[20] also described that the number of perforators is less compared with the other major blood vessels of the lower extremity. The diameters of the perforators have been correlated with number and size of branches to the fascial plexus. Some of these distal perforators do not give off any branches to the fascial plexus. The skin on the lateral side of the leg is therefore not totally dependent on the cutaneous perforating vessels from the peroneal artery. In a study by Ozlap and colleagues,[22] 9 cadavers were used to map out the perforator distribution relative to location and in designing a flap. There were 4 to 7 perforators shown in oblique projections from posterior to anterior and distal to proximal because of the course of the intramuscular septum between the peroneus longus and the soleus muscle. The lower, most septocutaneous perforator was 1.7 cm away from the posterior margin of the fibula. The upper, most septocutaneous perforator was 0.25 cm from the posterior fibular ridge.

Surgical Technique

Perioperatively, a handheld Doppler probe should be used in order to locate the peroneal artery and the most appropriate perforator vessel based on the given wound. The patient is to be placed in a supine position. A thigh tourniquet is placed for hemostasis control and the hip is bumped in order to gain exposure to the lateral aspect of the leg and subsequently the wound for flap coverage. Before prep, the extremity appears as

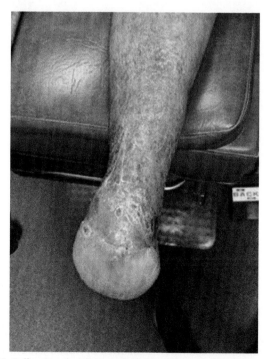

Fig. 6. Case study 1. Following development of a health granular base, a split-thickness skin graft was applied. At this time, the patient issue is resolved, and the wound remains healed. (*Courtesy of* R. Fahim DPM, Warren, OH.)

pictured. After adequate soft tissue debridement of the wound, the outline of the flap should be drawn based on defect size and shape in order to ensure enough donor site is harvested to cover the recipient site. Flap dissection should begin anteriorly to the subfascial layer, continuing dorsal and to the posterior side. This dissection is performed until the septocutaneous perforator or musculocutaneous perforator is visible and identified. The raised flap should be able to rotate around the perforator without any kinking of the perforator sacrificing the perfusion. The donor site in primarily closed under little tension and the recipient site is covered with the freshly harvested graft and sutured to the edges of the surgically debrided wound. In some cases, a split-thickness skin graft can be done in conjunction with the graft; however, the authors prefer to wait several days to ensure that the graft takes to the wound bed.

Our first case is a 61-year-old male patient who presented with gas gangrene extending into his midfoot. Initially, a surgical decompression, incision and drainage, and guillotine amputation at the level of the Chopart joint was performed. Following medical stabilization, thorough vascular work-up and consultation with an infectious disease specialist was conducted and the patient was determined to be an adequate candidate for peroneal adipofascial transfer. **Fig. 1** shows the wound before surgical intervention. The harvest was performed as previously described. Primary closure of the donor site from the lateral aspect of the leg followed harvest of the adipofascial

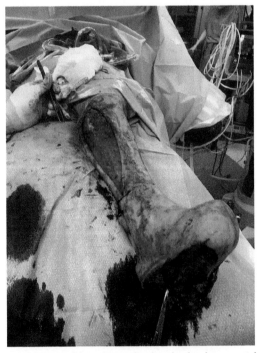

Fig. 7. Case study 2. A 50-year-old patient who has had subsequent heel ulceration and repeated wound infection following a transmetatarsal amputation a year earlier. This patient was treated with incision and drainage, lavage, and application of negative pressure vacuum wound therapy. This treatment was followed by wound care and hyperbaric oxygen therapy, which has resulted in failure of closure of the wound. A large plantar wound to the foot can be seen following debridement and exposure of the peroneal subcutaneous layer. (*Courtesy of* R. Fahim DPM, Warren, OH.)

flap and placing a drain (**Fig. 2**). The harvested flap is shown in order to demonstrate length and coverage of the medial aspect of the amputation site where there was exposed bone (**Figs. 3** and **4**). At this time, once the harvest was secured, a dermal matrix was used for coverage of the adipofascial flap in order to stimulate granulation tissue for the recipient skin graft to be planned in the near future (**Fig. 5**). At this time, an external fixator was placed in order to stabilize the graft while the wound healed in order to prevent any shearing forces from the ankle joint range of motion that would result in failure. **Fig. 6** shows the final result after obtaining a healthy granular base and harvest and application of a split-thickness skin graft. The patient remains healed at the time of publication.

The second case involves a 50-year-old patient (**Fig. 7**) who developed heel ulceration with repeated wound infection following a transmetatarsal amputation a year prior. This patient was treated with incision and drainage, lavage, and application of negative pressure vacuum wound therapy. This treatment was followed by wound care and hyperbaric oxygen therapy, which has resulted in failure of closure of the wound. A large plantar wound to the foot remained following debridement and exposure of the peroneal subcutaneous layer. **Fig. 8** shows harvest of the adipofascial flap and primary closure of the harvest site. The transfer of the flap is shown in **Figs. 9** and **10**. The flap was laid down in a turnover technique over intact skin. Following take of this graft, the bridge was resected, and the remaining primary harvest site was closed. The adipofascial transfer was then covered with a dermal matrix and further allowed to granulate. On the third visit to the operating room, a split-thickness skin graft was used to obtain definitive closure of the wound.

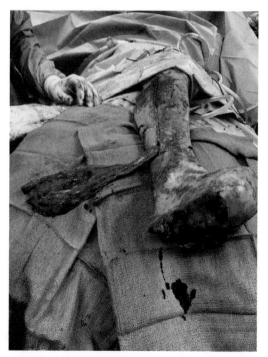

Fig. 8. Case study 2. Harvest of the adipofascial flap and primary closure of the harvest site. The arc of rotation can be seen. (*Courtesy of* R. Fahim DPM, Warren, OH.)

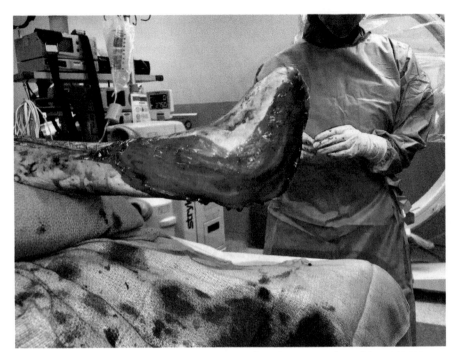

Fig. 9. Case study 2. The placement of the harvest flap. (*Courtesy of* R. Fahim DPM, Warren, OH.)

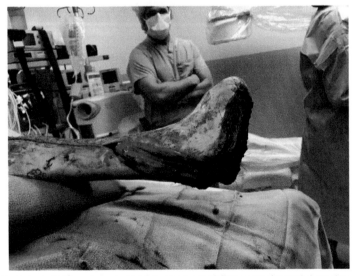

Fig. 10. Case study 2. The placement of the harvested flap onto the recipient site. (*Courtesy of* R. Fahim DPM, Warren, OH.)

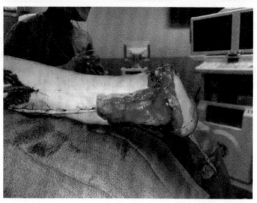

Fig. 11. Case study 3. A 42-year-old female patient who underwent an open Syme amputation at the ankle for a necrotizing fasciitis. There was not enough soft tissue for closure so it was determined from vascular assessment that the patient was an adequate candidate for adipofascial flap. Adipofascial flap was harvested in similar fashion as described earlier and applied to the lateral and anterior aspect of the distal lower extremity. (*Courtesy of* R. Fahim DPM, Warren, OH.)

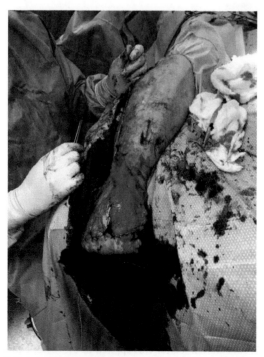

Fig. 12. Case study 3. Extremity before flap remodeling and transfer for a Syme amputation. (*Courtesy of* R. Fahim DPM, Warren, OH.)

The third case involves a 42-year-old female patient who underwent an open Syme amputation at the ankle for a necrotizing fasciitis. There was not enough soft tissue for closure so it was determined from vascular assessment that the patient was an adequate candidate for adipofascial flap. Adipofascial flap was harvested in similar fashion as described earlier and applied to the anterior and lateral aspects of the distal lower extremity (**Figs. 11** and **12**). An external fixator was applied to the lower extremity to protect the flap throughout the healing process through offloading (**Figs. 13–16**).

Bekara and colleagues[8] showed in a 2016 study that there are certain risk factors that show a direct correlation with flap failure. Patients with diabetes, aged more than 60 years, and with peripheral vascular disease should be approached with caution and should be medically and nutritionally optimized before intervention. In addition to this, the ratio of harvested flap length to width plays an important role in the flap's survival, particularly the distal aspect of the flap.[23] Lin and colleagues[24] stressed potential failure with not only the length/width ratio but also the flap-area/base-area ratio. Failure of the flap can occur in some cases, either partial or complete, and can also be the result of technical error. In a study by Chiu and colleagues,[25] fasciocutaneous flaps were deemed to be more significantly associated with flap failure and recurrence rate than myocutaneous and perforator flaps in paraplegic patients.

Postoperative Course for Lower Extremity Adipofascial Flaps

Following flap mobilization and donor site closure, and potentially application of an external fixator, a nonadherent dressing is applied to the flap and a bulky dressing

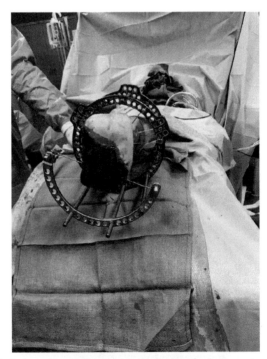

Fig. 13. Case study 3. An external fixator was applied to the lower extremity to protect the flap throughout the healing process through offloading. (*Courtesy of* R. Fahim DPM, Warren, OH.)

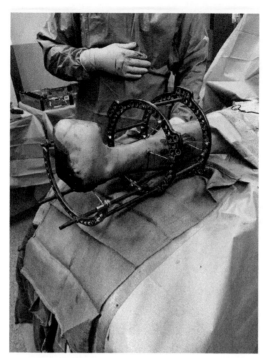

Fig. 14. Case study 3. An external fixator was applied to the lower extremity to protect the flap throughout the healing process through offloading. This view is from an alternate angle. (*Courtesy of* R. Fahim DPM, Warren, OH.)

is applied. Care of the local flap requires close observation to detect potential complications and early flap failure. Kerrigan and colleagues[26] reviewed various techniques for subjective assessment of flap viability and noted that color, capillary blanching, and warmth were unreliable indicators of viability. They found that bleeding from a puncture of the flap is likely the most accurate to clinically assess the flap's health.[26] Patients should be held on bed rest with elevated extremity to offload the limb. External fixation can assist in offloading if the flap recipient site is on the posterior aspect of the extremity. To better optimize this patient population, the authors recommend that patients be admitted to a skilled nursing facility in order to receive appropriate antibiotics, be optimized medically, and have ease of access in monitoring them.

The flap must be monitored early and often for any complications. In the first 24 hours, there is reduction in the arterial blood supply for the first 12 hours, which that begins to reverse at this point, leading to potential edema and congestion at the 24-hour mark. Prevention of vasospasm is of the utmost important in the early postoperative period. Edema is a concern, because it presents a large risk relative to the viability of the flap. The dressing should not prevent venous outflow, which would result in congestion of the harvested graft. If venous congestion is a concern, sutures must be removed from the flap where there is tension. Throughout the postoperative period, the flap is monitored for color, congestion, and evidence of flap failure. Between 48 and 72 hours, dressings should be removed, and, if drains are used, they can be removed during this phase if there are vascular anastomoses between the flap and the recipient bed forming. At 3 days to 1 week, there is progressive increase in

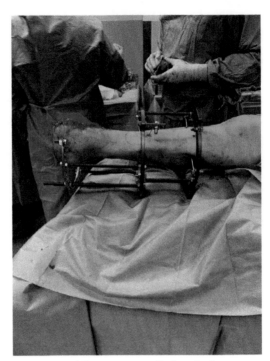

Fig. 15. Case study 3. An external fixator was applied to the lower extremity to protect the flap throughout the healing process through offloading. This view is from an alternate angle. (*Courtesy of* R. Fahim DPM, Warren, OH.)

the circulation of the flap, reaching a plateau at the 7-day mark. At this point, there is an increase in the number and caliber of longitudinal anastomoses and increase in numbers of small vessels in the pedicle. From this point, the vascular supply of the recipient bed increases, plateauing at 2 weeks and progressing to normalization and maturation within weeks 3 and 4 respectively. In the third week, the flap has developed most of its final circulation.[27]

Prevention of desiccation of ischemic tissue at the flap edges can help to prevent tissue loss. The temperature and blood flow of the flaps are important; and colder temperatures can cause constriction and increased blood viscosity, whereas warmth can result in the opposite. Hussal and colleagues[28] found that blood flow reduced from 65% of baseline in O_2 consumption when cooled to 20°C to 25% of baseline.

The patient's nicotine status also has an effect on wound healing and viability of the flap. Forrest and colleagues[29] described the effects of nicotine on capillary blood flow in rat models, showing significantly decreased capillary blood flow, perfusion, and flap survivability.

Complications

Venous congestion is the most common complication of fasciocutaneous and adipofascial flaps. Although peroneal artery flaps have excellent arterial perfusion, as previously discussed, flap edema caused by venous insufficiency can cause pressure necrosis to the flap. To minimize this complication, understanding the venous network and optimization of venous return can prevent flap complications being frequently encountered. With the turn-down approach, there is concern about the vein becoming

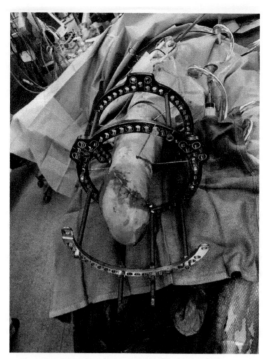

Fig. 16. Case study 3. An external fixator was applied to the lower extremity to protect the flap throughout the healing process through offloading. This view is from an alternate angle. (*Courtesy of* R. Fahim DPM, Warren, OH.)

kinked and contributing to significant flap edema. If this is suspected postoperatively, turning the flap back and staging transposition can resolve significant acute venous congestion. Warm saline, papaverine or nitroglycerin paste, and leech therapy have all been shown to be helpful for flap venous congestion.[30] Negative pressure wound therapy is controversial and should be used at low settings if considered.[31]

CLINICAL CARE POINTS

- The peroneal artery adipofascial flap is a useful workhorse for coverage of defects on the posterolateral aspect of the distal one-third of the leg.
- A thorough noninvasive vascular assessment must be performed and, if necessary, referral should be made for intervention before consideration of surgical intervention.
- Intraoperative use of Doppler is helpful in order to determine locations of the flap's perforators approximately 6 to 10 cm above the lateral malleolus.
- Following harvest and transfer of the adipofascial flap, it is imperative that a care team monitors the patient carefully in order to create the ideal environment for take of the graft and prevention of failure.
- Leg elevation and warming of the extremity should be encouraged to prevent edema and congestion of the flap. The authors recommend placement of the patient into a skilled nursing facility or a long-term acute care rehabilitation center in order to have control of external factors that may delay or impair the healing process.

DISCLOSURE

None.

REFERENCES

1. Cheng L, Yang X, Chen T, et al. Peroneal artery perforator flap for the treatment of chronic lower extremity wounds. J Orthop Surg Res 2017;12:170.
2. Mathes SJ, Nahai F. Reconstructive surgery: principles, anatomy & technique, vol. 2. New York: Churchill Livingstone; 1997. St. Louis: Quality Medical.
3. Gottlieb LJ, Krieger LM. From the reconstructive ladder to the reconstructive elevator. Plast Reconstr Surg 1994;93:1503–4.
4. Wong CJ, Niranjan N. Reconstructive stages as an alternative to the reconstructive ladder. Plast Reconstr Surg 2008;121:362e–3e.
5. Janis JE, Kwon RK, Attinger CE. The new reconstructive ladder: modifications to the traditional model. Plastic and Reconstructive Surgery 2011;127:205S–12S.
6. Nanda D, Anand Sahu S, Karki D, et al. Adipofascial perforator flaps: its role in reconstruction of soft-tissue defects of lower leg and ankle. Indian J Plast Surg 2018;51(2):216–21.
7. Lee S, Estela CM, Burd A. The lateral distally based adipofascial flap of the lower limb. Br J Plast Surg 2001;54:303–9.
8. Bekara F, Herlin C, Mojallal A, et al. A systematic review and meta-analysis of perforator-pedicled propeller flaps in lower extremity defects. Plast Reconstr Surg 2016;137(1):314–31.
9. Lai CS, Lin SD, Chou CK, et al. Clinical application of adipofascial turn-over flaps for burn wounds. Burns 1993;19:73–6.
10. Lee KJ, Lee SH, Kim MB, et al. Adipofascial fold-down flaps based on the posterior tibial artery perforator to cover the medial foot and ankle defects. J Plast Reconstr Aesthet Surg 2016;69(12):e229–37.
11. Buono P, Castus P, Dubois-Ferrière V, et al. Muscular versus non-muscular free flaps for soft tissue coverage of chronic tibial osteomyelitis. World J Plast Surg 2018;7(3):294–300.
12. Tahsin OG, Acartu€rk UZ, Tunc S, et al. Versatility of the perforator-based adipose, adipofascial, and fasciocutaneous flaps in reconstruction of distal leg and foot defects. J Foot Ankle Surg 2016. https://doi.org/10.1053/j.jfas.2014.12.020.
13. Cavadas PC, Sanz-Giménez-Rico JR, Gutierrez-de la Cámara A, et al. The medial sural artery perforator free flap. Plast Reconstr Surg 2001;108(6):1609–17.
14. Schmidt K, Zahn RK, Waschke J, et al. Subfascial directionality of perforators of the distal lower extremity: an anatomic study regarding selection of perforators for 180-degree propeller flaps. Ann Plast Surg 2012;69(3):307–11.
15. Paro J, Chiou G, Sen SK. Comparing muscle and fasciocutaneous free flaps in lower extremity reconstruction—does it matter? Ann Plast Surg 2016;76:S213–5.
16. Yoshimura M, Imura S, Shimamura K, et al. Peroneal flap for reconstruction in the extremity: preliminary report. Plast Reconstr Surg 1984;74(3):402–9.
17. Lin SD, Lai CS, Chou CK, et al. Reconstruction of soft tissue defects of the lower leg with the distally based medial adipofascial flap. Br J Plast Surg 1994;47:132–7.
18. Li B, Shi-Min C, Shou-Chao D, et al. Distally based sural adipofascial turnover flap for coverage of complicated wound in the foot and ankle region. Ann Plast Surg 2019;84(5):580–7.

19. Purushothaman R, Balakrishnan TM, Alalasundaram KV. Anatomical study of terminal peroneal artery perforators and their clinical applications Indian. J Plast Surg 2013;46(1):69–74.
20. Batchelor JS, Moss AL. The relationship between fasciocutaneous perforators and their fascial branches: an anatomical study in human cadaver lower legs. Plast Reconstr Surg 1995. https://doi.org/10.1097/00006534-199504000-00001.
21. KM Robertson, LRCSI, LRCPI, FACS. Fasciocutaneous Flaps Medscape Updated: May 06, 2019.
22. Ozalp T, Masquelet AC, Begue TC. Septocutaneous perforators of the peroneal artery relative to the fibula: anatomical basis of the use of pedicled fasciocutaneous flap. Surg Radiol Anat 2006;28(1):54–8.
23. Cai L, Huang W, Lin D. Effects of traditional Chinese medicine Shuxuetong injection on random skin flap survival in rats. ScientificWorldJournal 2014;2014: 816545.
24. Lin SD, Lai CS, Tsai CC, et al. Clinical application of the distally based medial adipofascial flap for soft tissue defects on the lower half of the leg. J Trauma 1995; 38:623–9.
25. Chiu YJ, Liao WC, Wang TH, et al. A retrospective study: multivariate logistic regression analysis of the outcomes after pressure sores reconstruction with fasciocutaneous, myocutaneous, and perforator flaps. J Plast Reconstr Aesthet Surg 2017;70(8):1038–43.
26. Kerrigan CL, Daniel RK. Skin flap research: a candid view. Ann Plast Surg 1984; 13:383.
27. Hoopes JE. Pedicle flaps—an overview. In: Krizek TJ, Hoopes JE, editors. Symposium on basic science in plastic surgery, vol. 15. St Louis (MO): Mosby; 1976. p. 241–59. Ch 28.
28. Hussl H, Guy RJ, Eriksson E, et al. Effect of temperature on blood flow and metabolism in a neurovascular island skin flap. Ann Plast Surg 1986;17:73.
29. Forrest CR, Xu N, Pang CY. Evidence for nicotine-induced skin flap ischemic necrosis in the pig. Can J Physiol Pharmacol 1994;72(1):30–8.
30. Yun MH, Sik Yoon E, Lee B-Il, et al. The effect of low-dose nitroglycerin ointment on skin flap necrosis in breast reconstruction after skin-sparing or nipple-sparing Mastectomy. Arch Plast Surg 2017;44(6):509–15.
31. Yu P, Yu N, Yang X, et al. Clinical efficacy and safety of negative-pressure wound therapy on flaps: a systematic review. J Reconstr Microsurg 2017; 33(5):358–66.

The Reverse Sural Artery Flap

A Reliable and Versatile Flap for Wound Coverage of the Distal Lower Extremity and Hindfoot

Lance Johnson, DPM[a], Michael D. Liette, DPM[a],
Chris Green, DPM[b,1], Pedro Rodriguez, MD[c],
Suhail Masadeh, DPM[d,*]

KEYWORDS

- Flap • Fasciocutaneous • Traumatic defect • Adipofascial
- Lower limb reconstruction

KEY POINTS

- The reverse sural artery flap is a stable and reliable option for soft tissue coverage of the distal lower extremity, ankle, and the posterior heel.
- The reverse sural artery flap has a short operative time with minimal donor site morbidity.
- The reverse sural artery flap provides an excellent gliding surface for exposed tendons.
- The reverse sural artery flap is used for coverage of exposed vessels, tendons, bones, and hardware.
- Venous congestion is the most common complication impacting flap success.

INTRODUCTION

Acute and chronic soft tissue defects of the distal lower extremity pose a significant challenge to the reconstructive surgeon. The paucity of vascularized tissue coupled with the mechanical demands of the region creates unique barriers in wound

[a] University of Cincinnati Medical Center, 231 Albert Sabin Way, ML 0513, Cincinnati, OH 45276, USA; [b] American College of Foot and Ankle Surgeons, Integris Limb Salvage Center, Oklahoma City, OK, USA; [c] Plastic and Reconstructive Surgery, OSF Saint Anthony Medical Center, University of Illinois, 698 Featherstone Road, Rockford, IL 61107, USA; [d] University of Cincinnati Medical Center, Cincinnati Veteran Affairs Medical Center, 231 Albert Sabin Way, ML 0513, Cincinnati, OH 45276, USA
[1] Present address: 13100 North Western Avenue, Suite 200 131, Oklahoma City, OK 73114.
* Corresponding author.
E-mail address: masadesb@uc.edu

Clin Podiatr Med Surg 37 (2020) 699–726
https://doi.org/10.1016/j.cpm.2020.05.004
0891-8422/20/Published by Elsevier Inc.

podiatric.theclinics.com

management. Advancements in microsurgery techniques and low complication rates have made free tissue transfer the treatment of choice for soft tissue coverage in the distal lower extremity.[1] However, because of the complexity of microsurgery and limited availability in some settings, the use of local pedicled flaps remains a viable alternative in select patients. The reverse sural artery flap (RSAF) provides a local option that is both versatile and reliable for covering soft tissue defects of the lower extremity.

The RSAF was originally described as a fasciocutaneous flap by Donski and Fogdestam[2,3] in 1983 and later popularized by Masquelet and colleagues in 1992. Since the original description, the RSAF has been relabeled with various modifications and nomenclature generating confusion throughout the literature. Several classifications of the flap are included in **Table 1**. Despite these various complications, the flap originates from the sural angiosome and has become a mainstay in the reconstruction of the lower extremity, ankle, and the posterior heel.[1]

REVERSE SURAL ARTERY FLAP ANATOMY

Since the original description by Donski and Fogdestam,[3] the RSAF has been studied extensively to explore the retrograde arterial supply, its relation to the sural nerve, and its venous drainage. The posterior lower extremity is supplied by the sural angiosome created by the medial and lateral sural arteries. The sural angiosome, created from the medial and lateral sural arteries, supplies the skin and fascia of the posterior lower extremity (**Fig. 1**). The sural angiosome is a dense arterial network of 1 to 3 musculocutaneous arteries named the medial, the median, and the lateral superficial sural arteries or sural cutaneous arteries. The median superficial sural artery (MSSA) is the largest, measuring 0.9 to 2.6 mm in diameter. The MSSA exits the popliteal fossa and travels between the 2 heads of the gastrocnemius muscle. Proximally, the artery is subfascial, becoming superficial at the level of the gastrocnemius musculotendinous junction, and is located medial to the lesser saphenous vein at the level of the lateral malleolus.[4-7]

The sural cutaneous arteries and the musculocutaneous perforators provide the anterograde flow for the sural angiosome. Historically, the blood supply of the reverse

Table 1	
These classifications of the reverse sural artery flap are often based on the surgical technique and the tissues included in the flap during harvest	
Name/Variation	**Authors**
Reverse sural artery flap	Price, Hong
Delayed sural flap	Kneser
Supercharged reverse sural flap	Tan
Sural fasciomusculocutaneous flap	Chen
Distally based sural flap	Follmar, Aoki
Cross-leg distally based sural flap	Eser
Distally based sural neurocutaneous flap	Hasegawa
Distally based sural neuro-fasciomyocutaneous flap	Chang
Distally based sural neuro-lesser saphenous veno-fasciocutaneous compound flap	Zhang
Nerve-sparing distally based sural fasciocutaneous flap	Aydin

Data from Refs.[1,13,22,26,27,30,37,38,41,50-52]

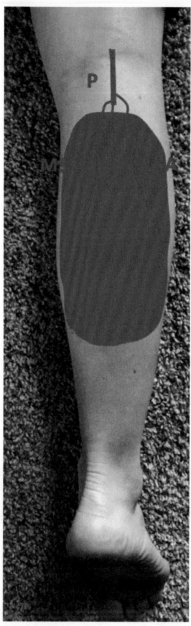

Fig. 1. The popliteal artery (P) branches into the medial (MSA) and lateral (LSA) sural arteries to help form the sural angiosome of the posterior leg. (*Courtesy of* S. Masadeh, DPM, Cincinnati, OH.)

sural flap is credited to the septocutaneous perforator of the peroneal artery. However, multiple anatomic studies established that the blood supply is based on 4 sources of perforators. This retrograde flow to the median sural artery is supplied by the peroneal artery septocutaneous perforators, the posterior tibial artery septocutaneous perforators, the lesser saphenous venocutaneous perforators, and the sural nerve neurocutaneous perforators.[7–9]

Within the lateral lower extremity, 3 to 6 peroneal artery septocutaneous perforators can be found. These perforators are fundamental when planning fasciocutaneous flaps in lower extremity reconstruction. The peroneal artery perforators provide vascular supply to the peroneal fasciocutaneous flap, the distally based peroneus brevis muscle flap, and the fibula when used as a vascularized autologous bone graft (**Fig. 2**).[4,7] The distal perforators additionally connect to the superficial sural arteries, providing retrograde flow for the RSAF flap. The most distal peroneal perforator is located 5 to 7 cm proximal to the tip of the lateral malleolus, at the midline between the fibular shaft and the Achilles.[1] Classically, the distal perforator serves as the pivot point for the rotation of the flap. However, there are reports of flap extension based on more distal perforators that allow coverage of the midfoot and the forefoot.[1,10]

The posterior tibial artery lies in the deep posterior compartment of the leg and provides 4 to 5 septocutaneous perforators to the medial lower extremity. Similar to the peroneal artery, the posterior tibial artery septocutaneous perforators supply their own fasciocutaneous flap as well as retrograde flow to the RSAF. The most distal septocutaneous perforator is located 4 and 10 cm proximal to the tip of the medial malleolus[4,5,11] (**Fig. 3**).

The lesser saphenous vein and the sural nerve augment the blood supply of the RSAF. The vasa vasorum and vasa nervorum provide the intrinsic blood supply of the vein and the nerve as well as the skin via neurocutaneous and venocutaneous perforators, respectively. The intrinsic and extrinsic blood supply is supported by loose areolar tissue often referred to as the mesentery (**Fig. 4**). It is important to avoid injury to this friable connective tissue and to ensure inclusion within the flap.[12]

The lesser saphenous vein aids in venous return of the distal lower extremity. The course begins at the lateral border of the dorsum of the foot and passes below the

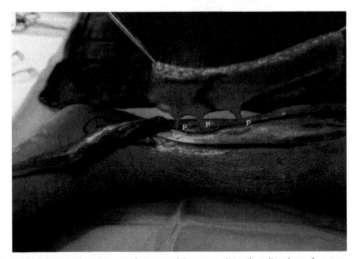

Fig. 2. Multiple peroneal artery perforators (P). Note that the distal perforator can supply the peroneal fasciocutaneous, distally based peroneus brevis, and the RSAF. (*Courtesy of* S. Masadeh, DPM, Cincinnati, OH.)

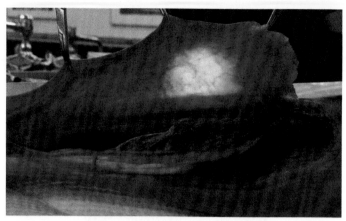

Fig. 3. Multiple perforators (P) of the posterior tibial artery, which contribute to the supply of the sural angiosome. (*Courtesy of* S. Masadeh, DPM, Cincinnati, OH.)

lateral malleolus. The vein travels along the posterior border of the fibula crossing the sural nerve at the distal one-third of the leg. More proximally, the lesser saphenous vein is located between the 2 heads of the gastrocnemius muscle. It is important to note that the lesser saphenous vein remains superficial to the deep fascia until it passes through the popliteal fossa to drain into the popliteal vein[12–15] **(Fig. 5)**. The orthograde valves within the lesser saphenous vein promote venous drainage and prevent reflux into the extremity. When the RSAF is rotated, the valves act as a barrier to retrograde flow and contribute to venous congestion. Because of the restriction of venous outflow, the flaps mechanism for venous return is through the venae comitantes.[1,12]

The sural nerve proper is formed by the union of the medial sural cutaneous nerve and the lateral sural cutaneous nerve (also known as the peroneal communicating branch). The sural nerve proper is often a continuation of the medial sural cutaneous nerve. The medial cutaneous sural nerve courses between the MSSA and the lesser

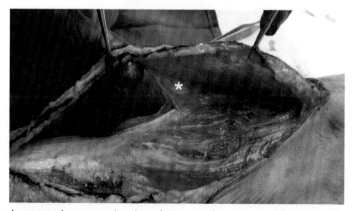

Fig. 4. The loose aerolar connective tissue known as the mesentery (*asterisk*). (*Courtesy of* P. Rodriguez, MD, Rockford, IL.)

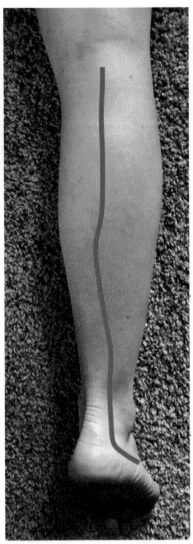

Fig. 5. The course of the lesser saphenous vein, at the proximal-most aspect, as it travels from the superficial fascia to the deep fascia in the popliteal fossa. (*Courtesy of* S. Masadeh, DPM, Cincinnati, OH.)

saphenous vein. It pierces the deep fascia after connecting with the lateral cutaneous sural nerve to become the sural nerve proper. The sural nerve proper travels along with the lesser saphenous vein and median sural artery. In the distal leg, the sural nerve is located between the MSSA and the Achilles tendon.[16,17] The RSAF is often referred to as the medial sural cutaneous flap. Union of the medial sural cutaneous nerve and the lateral sural cutaneous nerve does not occur 33% of the time (**Fig. 6**).[18–21]

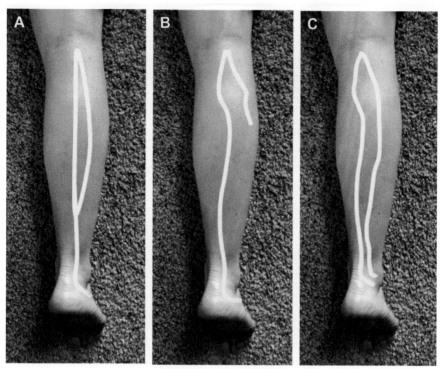

Fig. 6. The most common sural nerve variations: variations (*A*), (*B*), and (*C*) of the medial and lateral sural cutaneous nerves. (*A*) Combined pattern, which is the most common (72.5%). (*B*) The second most common (diminished) (17.5%). (*C*) The least common (10.0%).[21] (*Courtesy of* S. Masadeh, DPM, Cincinnati, OH.)

SURGICAL TECHNIQUE

The RSAF has multiple modifications and can be harvested as an adipofascial or as a fasciocutaneous flap; the latter is described here. The patient is placed in the prone position on the operating table after induction of general or regional anesthesia. The peroneal perforators are identified and outlined using a handheld Doppler. The posterior aspect of the fibula and the medial crest of the tibia are outlined and serve as the borders for the medial and lateral extensions (**Fig. 7**). A line is also drawn from the popliteal fossa to the midline of the Achilles tendon, serving as the flap axis. The superior margin of the flap is delineated by palpating the conjoined gastrocnemius heads proximally, and the inferior portion of the flap is delineated by a distinct separation distally. The gastrocnemius muscle is palpated, which is conjoined proximally, with a distinct separation distally. The cleavage point between the muscle heads is identified as the landmark for the location of the pedicle. The flap pivot point is then identified approximately 5 cm superior to the lateral malleolus. Pedicle length is determined by the distance of the pivot point to the nearest point of the defect. A proximal skin island is mapped to match the defect site according to the length necessary with the pedicle centralized. Saline solution may be injected subcutaneously and subfascial surrounding the area of the flap (**Fig. 8**). The main author infiltrates the site with saline solution to aid with flap elevation and dissection.

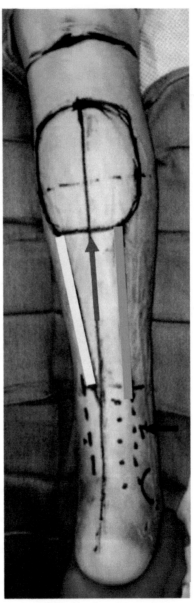

Fig. 7. Preoperative markings of the RSAF: a line is drawn from the popliteal fossa to the midline of the Achilles tendon, serving as the flap axis, and also corresponds to the cleavage point of the gastrocnemius muscle heads (*red arrow*). The skin paddle is drawn to match the defect. The lateral line (*green line*) represents the posterior aspect of the fibula, and the medial line (*yellow line*) represents the medial border of the tibia. The pivot point is located 7 cm from the tip of the lateral malleolus (*black arrow*). (*Courtesy of* S. Masadeh, DPM, Cincinnati, OH.)

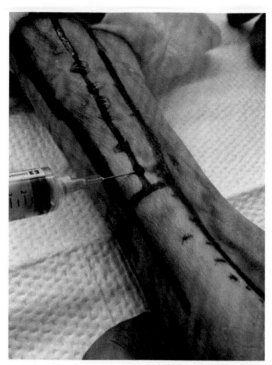

Fig. 8. Local anesthetic or saline is injected to separate the dermal-subdermal complex to facilitate dissection of the skin over the pedicle. Care should be taken to avoid direct infiltration of the flap in order to avoid injury to the pedicle. (*Courtesy of* S. Masadeh, DPM, Cincinnati, OH.)

The incision begins along the lateral border of the skin island, extending to the level of the deep fascia until the gastrocnemius muscle is identified. Care must be taken to avoid delamination of the skin island. Staples or sutures can be used to stabilize the deep fascia to the cutaneous construct. At the inferior margin of the skin island, the incision is made through the skin, avoiding violation of the subcutaneous tissue and injury to the pedicle. The incision is advanced in a midline fashion over the conjoined tendon again without violating the subcutaneous tissue. The skin is elevated from the subcutaneous tissue sharply with a number 10 blade, leaving a thin layer of subcutaneous fat attached to preserve the subdermal plexus of the skin and to avoid necrosis (**Fig. 9**). The skin is elevated medially and laterally to the previously outlined boarders. A 4-cm-wide pedicle should be maintained to optimize flap vascularity and venous drainage. Once the subcutaneous layer is exposed, a lateral fasciotomy is performed over the posterior border of the fibula, and the flap is elevated.

Although flap elevation has been traditionally performed in a proximal to distal fashion, the authors recommend elevating the flap from distal to proximal to the inferior aspect of the gastrocnemius muscle. This technique developed by Dr Rodriguez preserves the pedicle intact and allows protection of the pedicle during flap elevation. It is important to note that the sural nerve transitions from subfascial to superficial fascia at the inferior portion and midline of the medial and lateral gastrocnemius heads (**Fig. 10**). At the transition zone, the pedicle is densely attached to the fascia. Elevating the flap from distal to proximal ensures reliability and reproducibility in identification of

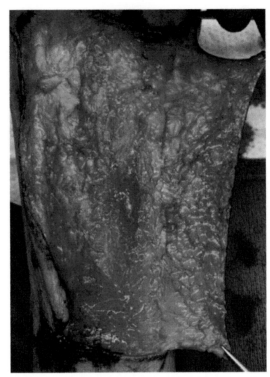

Fig. 9. Cobblestone appearance of the subcutaneous tissue and the dermis as it is reflected away from the fascia proper of the reverse sural flap, maintaining a layer of subdermal fat, decreases the risk of skin necrosis. (*Courtesy of* S. Masadeh, DPM, Cincinnati, OH.)

the pedicle (**Fig. 11**). Once the interface between the deep and superficial zones of the pedicle is identified, the island flap can be elevated from the gastrocnemius muscle (**Fig. 12**). To avoid injury to the mesentery of the neurovascular bundle, a 2-mm muscle cuff may be included in the flap to avoid violation of the mesentery. It is important to

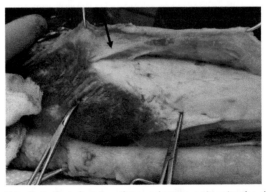

Fig. 10. Intraoperative dissection showing the sural nerve as it exits the deep fascia and enters the superficial fascia (*black arrow*). Note the location of the pedicle along the central raphe. (*Courtesy of* S. Masadeh, DPM, Cincinnati, OH.)

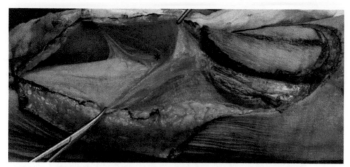

Fig. 11. Visualized is the elevation of the medial flap margins with identification of the pedicle. A retractor, often an Army-Navy, is used to lift the pedicle up as dissection is continued to ensure its incorporation within the flap margins. Note, the transition zone (*asterisk*), the pedicle transitions from loosely adhered to densely adhered to the underlying fascia. A distal to proximal dissection allows for reproducible inclusion of the pedicle. (*Courtesy of* S. Masadeh, DPM, Cincinnati, OH.)

maintain a sufficient length of the lesser saphenous vein with flap harvest in case flap "supercharging" is required.[22]

   The previously marked skin paddle is incised down to the deep fascia. Once the flap is elevated, the lesser saphenous vein is cannulized and injected with heparinized saline to remove any thrombi and promote venous drainage (**Figs. 13** and **14**). The flap is then rotated 180°, inset over the defect, and secured without tension (**Fig. 15**). The donor site is closed primarily or skin grafted pending the size of the defect. A drain is placed to allow for fluid drainage and help prevent hematoma or seroma formation. The limb is immobilized to prevent shearing forces that are detrimental to flap healing. Immobilization can be achieved via external fixation or a well-padded splint with a window for flap monitoring.

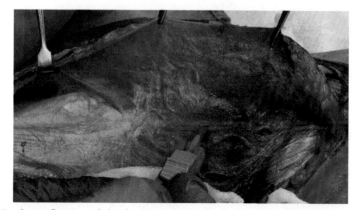

Fig. 12. Further reflection of the fasciocutaneous flap with clear delineation of superficial and deep zones. Inclusion of the mesentery is ensured by incorporating a small, 1-mm cuff of the gastrocnemius muscle to maximize flap perfusion. (*Courtesy of* S. Masadeh, DPM, Cincinnati, OH.)

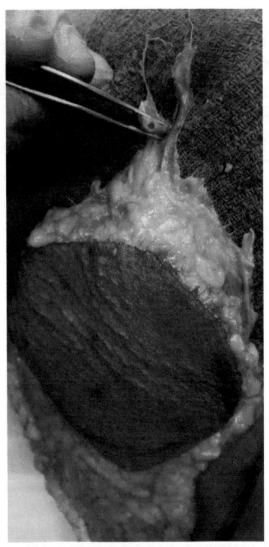

Fig. 13. A patent lesser saphenous vein is demonstrated in the figure. It is important to harvest an adequate length of the lesser saphenous vein that can be used for "supercharging" or cannulization of the flap. (*Courtesy of* S. Masadeh, DPM, Cincinnati, OH.)

REVERSE SURAL FLAP MODIFICATIONS

Modifications of the RSAF are based on the harvest technique or the tissue composition. The original description of the fasciocutaneous flap had up to a 70% complication rate because of venous congestion.[23–25] The flap was originally described with a 2-cm-wide pedicle. Sugg and colleagues[25] popularized the 4-cm-wide pedicle. In addition, they discussed having an adipofascial pedicle or a fasciocutaneous skin bridge. Transitioning to a 4-cm-wide pedicle decreased the venous congestion by capturing additional veins within the pedicle to improve venous drainage (**Fig. 16**). Lee and

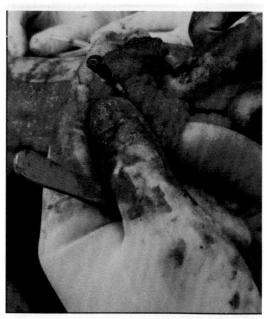

Fig. 14. An angiocatheter is placed into the lesser saphenous vein in order to cannulize the vein. Heparinized saline can be flushed through the angiocatheter in order to remove thrombi within the vein. (*Courtesy of* S. Masadeh, DPM, Cincinnati, OH.)

colleagues[10] discussed leaving a skin extension on the pedicle (**Fig. 17**A–G). They theorized the skin extension over the pedicle reduced complications by avoiding compression of the pedicle and increasing reach of the flap.

The reversal of flow in the lesser saphenous vein after rotation increases venous congestion. The "supercharging" technique decreases congestion by anastomosing the lesser saphenous vein to a local vein.[22] The anastomosis restores physiologic flow, improving drainage of the flap. However, this requires microvenous anastomosis and the presence of an adequate local vein. An alternative to supercharging is catheterization of the lesser saphenous vein, allowing for periodic drainage of the flap.[1] Last, the lesser saphenous vein can be ligated at the distal aspect of the lateral malleolus to prevent reflux into the flap.[1,26,27]

Another technical modification to improve perfusion is delaying of the flap. Delay results in local vasodilation of the choke vessels; this is accomplished by complete flap elevation, with immediate return to the harvest site. Alternatively, the medial and lateral borders of the flap are incised, therefore maximizing longitudinal flow with subsequent complete harvest and inset 2 weeks later.[3,28–33] The length of delay has been discussed in several articles, but the senior authors' preferred time of delay is 14 days if possible to allow full dilatation of the venae comitantes.[3,28–33] When not possible to wait the full 2 weeks, the authors place a catheter for controlled drainage. Delaying the flap should be used if the superficial vein is absent or injured[34] (**Figs. 18–21**).

Another modification involves nerve-sparing or splitting techniques. Traditionally, the sural nerve is sacrificed during flap elevation to achieve adequate pedicle length.[21] Nerve sacrifice often leads to hypoesthesia along the sural nerve sensory distribution and stump neuroma formation.[35] The nerve-sparing technique involves dissection of

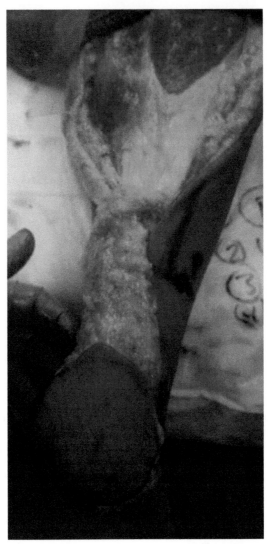

Fig. 15. Inset of a fasciocutaneous island flap to cover a posterior heel defect. (*Courtesy of* S. Masadeh, DPM, Cincinnati, OH.)

the sural nerve from the mesentery and exclusion from the flap (**Fig. 22**). Some investigators postulate that the sural nerve is not needed for flap survival and can be modified into a venocutaneous flap.[36–38] Nerve-splitting techniques involve the preservation of the medial sural cutaneous nerve. The medial and lateral nerves lie in different fascial planes with the lateral being more superficial before uniting to form the sural nerve proper. During flap harvest, the lateral sural cutaneous nerve is transected and split from the medial sural cutaneous nerve. The nerves are separated until sufficient length is acquired to cover the defect. This technique avoids neuroma formation while preserving sensation to the lateral leg and foot.[21]

The flap can be harvested as an adipofascial or myofasciocutaneous flap. When harvested without skin, it is known as an adipofascial flap. Excluding the skin has

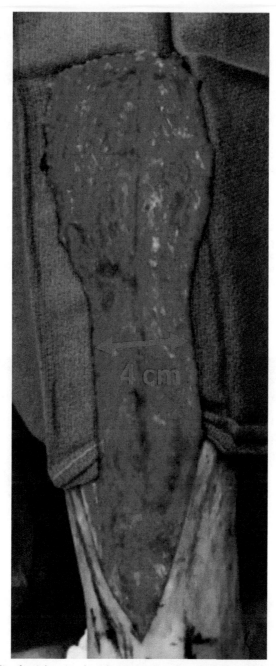

Fig. 16. RSAF (adipofascial variant) with 4-cm-wide adipofascial pedicle. (*Courtesy of* P. Rodriguez MD, Rockford, IL.)

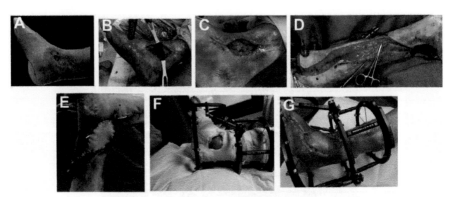

Fig. 17. (A–G) (A) Patient with a medial wound with exposed bone and a septic ankle joint. (B) The wound after debridement and resection of the ankle joint. (C) After resection of the ankle joint, the procedure is staged, and an antibiotic spacer is placed within the wound. (D, E) An RSAF (fasciocutaneous variant) with extended skin bridge along the pedicle (D) and subsequent inset of the flap (E). (F) Window dressing is placed so that the skin island is readily accessible to check for signs of venous congestion. The limb is stabilized with an external fixator. (G) The limb after incorporation and complete healing of the flap. (Courtesy of S. Masadeh, DPM, Cincinnati, OH.)

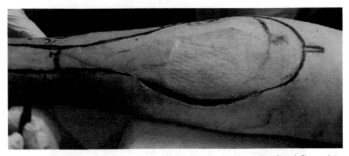

Fig. 18. The medial and lateral incisions made to maximize longitudinal flow. (Courtesy of S. Masadeh, DPM, Cincinnati, OH.)

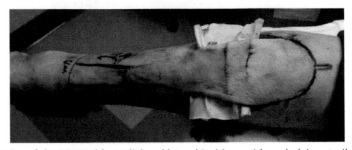

Fig. 19. Delay of the RSAF with medial and lateral incisions with underlying sterile powder-free glove. (Courtesy of S. Masadeh, DPM, Cincinnati, OH.)

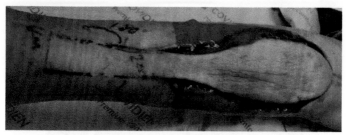

Fig. 20. Delay of the RSAF with medial and lateral incisions with underlying acellular dermal regenerative template. (*Courtesy of* S. Masadeh, DPM, Cincinnati, OH.)

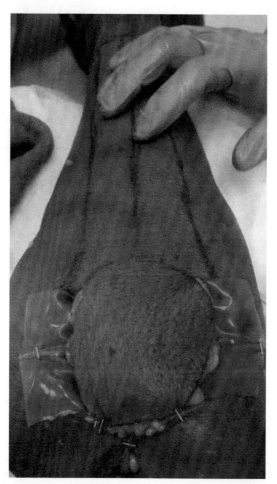

Fig. 21. Delay of the RSAF with medial, lateral, and proximal incisions with underlying acellular dermal regenerative template. (*Courtesy of* S. Masadeh, DPM, Cincinnati, OH.)

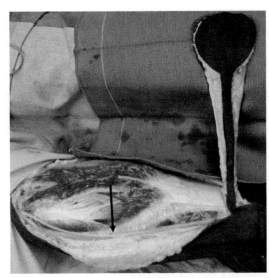

Fig. 22. Intraoperative nerve variant. Note that the lateral sural cutaneous nerve (*arrow*) is superficial and the medial sural cutaneous nerve is deep. A nerve-sparing technique can be used in a similar fashion by preserving the medial sural cutaneous nerve. (*Courtesy of* S. Masadeh, DPM, Cincinnati, OH.)

several advantages, such as decreasing the metabolic demand, increasing the reach, and allowing for primary closure of the donor site (**Fig. 23**). However, the flap requires a split-thickness skin graft[3,25] (**Fig. 24**). When harvested with a section of muscle, it is known as a myofasciocutaneous flap. The myofasciocutaneous variation involves harvesting a section of the gastrocnemius muscle along with the fascial component. The muscle provides increased bulk for deeper deficits and a protective layer for the pedicle (**Figs. 25** and **26**).[3,14,15] Furthermore, it is postulated that the musculocutaneous perforators provide additional vascularity to the RSAF.[39,40] The size of the muscle harvested is based on the incorporation of the musculocutaneous perforators, which is often one-third of either the medial or lateral gastrocnemius heads.[34,41,42]

LITERATURE REVIEW/RESULTS

Three systematic reviews evaluating RSAF patient demographics, outcomes, and complications have been isolated for review.[3,43,44] The findings are presented in **Table 2**.

ANALYSIS/DISCUSSION

Acute and chronic wounds of the lower extremity and hindfoot are challenging for the reconstructive surgeon. The RSAF has proven to be a reliable alternative to free tissue transfer in select patients.[1,43,45] The RSAF may be used to cover exposed, tendon, bone, hardware, or neurovascular structures (**Fig. 27**). The RSAF is commonly used for coverage of the posterior heel, including exposed Achilles tendon, and dehisced anterior ankle surgical incisions, such as those used for total ankle replacements.[44,46] Flap dissection does not require special instrumentation, extensive surgical experience, or specialized centers capable of stringent postoperative monitoring requirements in comparison to free flaps.[14,15] The procedure requires a relatively short

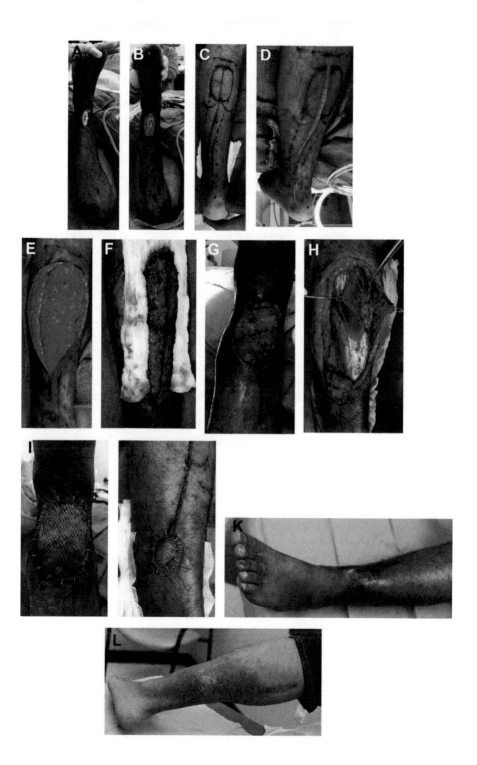

operative time compared with free flap harvest and does not sacrifice any major source artery to the foot. The flap has a wide arc of rotation with minimal donor site morbidity, particularly when using the adipofascial variant. The versatility of the RSAF allows for easy contouring to the posterior heel, which aids in shoe fit and bracing.[1,44,47,48]

Preoperative planning is critical for a successful outcome. In traumatic wounds, all osseous injuries must be stabilized. Medical optimization is essential for patients with multiple comorbidities. Acoustic or color Doppler examination is often sufficient to determine the vascular status of the operative limb; however, if there is concern for peroneal artery occlusion, advanced imaging is recommended. Aggressive debridement to remove all nonviable tissue and for the reduction of bacterial bioburden is the foundation for wound bed preparation and successful incorporation of the flap.[1,43,49]

Complication rates have wide ranges throughout the literature, of which most are minor and managed without a return to the operating room. Total flap necrosis rates range from 3% to 10%, which is comparable to free flap in lower limb reconstruction.[43] Partial flap necrosis rates are approximately 15%, similar again to that of the rates seen for free flaps of the lower limb.[30,44] Higher rates of partial and total flap loss are reported in patients with comorbidities, such as diabetes mellitus and peripheral vascular disease. In this cohort of patients, complication rates occur in up to 50% of cases, with 11.5% of patients suffering total flap loss. In a systematic review of 43 studies, Daar and colleagues[44] concluded that the rate of complete flap loss was comparable to the healthy population; however, they noted higher partial flap loss rates in patients with comorbidities. They also reported significantly increased rates of partial flap loss in patients who smoke. Regardless of health status, the most common complication of the RSAF is partial flap necrosis, often owing to venous congestion.

Modification of surgical technique, such as flap delay, supercharging, and a wide pedicle, has been reported to improve venous drainage. These techniques should be used in patients with venous insufficiency, diabetes mellitus, peripheral vascular disease, and smokers, as well as in cases with extended flap dimensions.[44]

In their systematic review and metaanalysis, Follmar and colleagues[1] analyzed the outcomes of the RSAF.[1] Of the flaps included in the review, 82% healed without complication. They noted a total flap loss of 3.3% and partial flap necrosis of 11%. Other complications experienced were noted to be recurrent infection, edema, and venous congestion. These complications were considered to be reasonable and readily manageable. Studies included in this metaanalysis

Fig. 23. (A–K) (A) A patient with exposed tibialis anterior tendon devoid of synovial sheath. (B) The wound bed after debridement. (C) The preoperative RSAF design with the course of the sural nerve outlined to ensure the incorporation within the flap after completion of elevation. (D) The incision for the adipofascial RSAF is made along the course of the sural nerve. (E) The skin is dissected from the underlying subcutaneous tissue. (F) Elevation of the flap with subsequent tunneling and (G) inset. (H) To decrease the chances of symptomatic stump formation, the residual medial sural cutaneous nerve is secured and buried between the medial and lateral gastrocnemius heads (neuromyodesis). (I, J) Skin grafting of the adipofascial flap and at the entrance to the subcutaneous tunnel. (K, L) A completely healed adipofascial RSAF. (*Courtesy of* P. Rodriguez MD, Rockford, IL.)

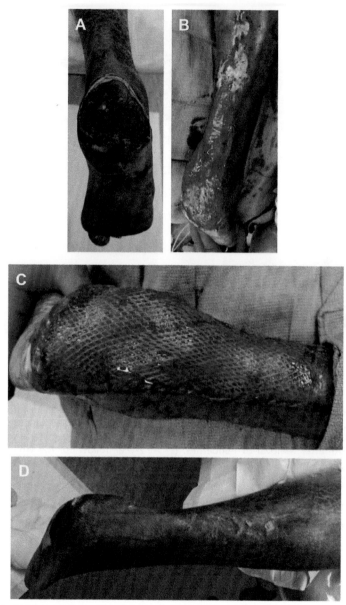

Fig. 24. (*A–D*) (*A*) A patient with necrotic heel ulceration. (*B*) Preparation of an adipofascial RSAF for a split-thickness skin graft. (*C*) An adipofascial RSAF with overlying split-thickness skin graft. (*D*) A completely healed split-thickness skin and RSAF. (*Courtesy of* S. Masadeh, DPM, Cincinnati, OH.)

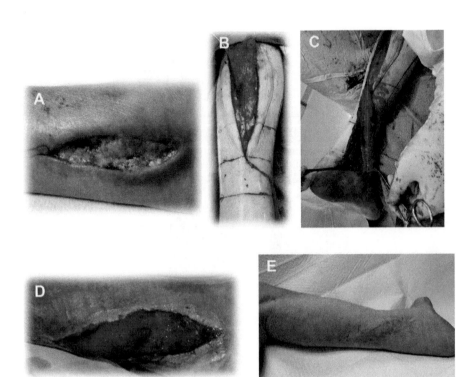

Fig. 25. (*A–E*) (*A*) A wound dehiscence with exposed vein graft after distal posterior tibial artery bypass graft for a patient with peripheral arterial disease. (*B*) The elevation of a myoadipofascial RSAF. (*C*) The myoadipofascial flap after harvest with a section of medial head of the gastrocnemius muscle. The flap was temporized with a dermal regenerative template. (*D*) The RSAF after removal of neodermis. (*E*) At 2-year follow-up, the wound remains healed with a cosmetically acceptable appearance. (*Courtesy of* S. Masadeh, DPM, Cincinnati, OH.)

were composed of young healthy patients; however, the investigators postulated that patients with multiple comorbidities would have a higher rate of complications.[1,25]

In conclusion, the RSAF provides a reliable local alternative for wound coverage of the distal lower extremity and hindfoot. The flap is based on the peroneal artery, posterior tibial artery, neurocutaneous, and venocutaneous perforators. The distal peroneal artery perforators, located 5 to 7 cm above the lateral malleolus, serve as the pivot point for the flap. Although higher complication rates are reported in the comorbid patient, the RSAF remains a reliable option in the management of these complex wounds. The surgeon must be familiar with the management techniques for venous congestion. The RSAF is a valuable option for the lower-extremity reconstructive surgeon.

CLINICAL CARE POINTS

- The RSAF can be used for soft tissue defects up to 10 × 12 cm in size.
- The RSAF pivot point is based on the distal peroneal artery perforator.

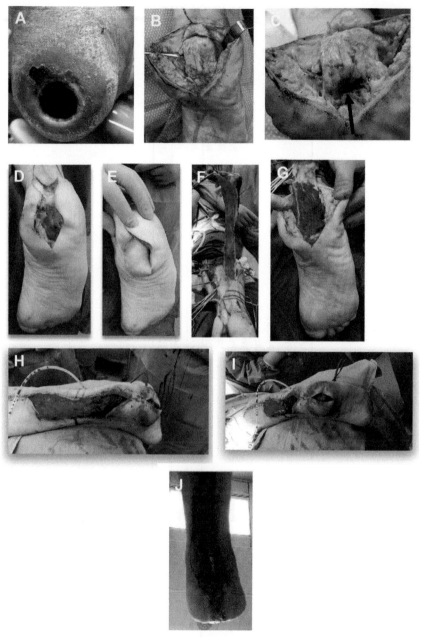

Fig. 26. (*A–J*) (*A*) A patient with diabetes mellitus and a plantar heel ulcer with osteomyelitis secondary to calcaneal gait. (*B*) Exposed calcaneus after wide excision of ulceration. (*C*) Calcaneal osteomyelitis with noted sinus tract. (*D*) The wound after partial calcanectomy. (*E*) After partial calcanectomy, there is notable dead space in the defect. In order to preserve the weight-bearing skin and contour of the heel, a myoadipofascial flap was used to fill the deficit. (*F*) An intraoperative photograph demonstrating surgical elevation of RSAF. (*G*) An intraoperative photograph demonstrating inset of RSAF. (*H*) RSAF after inset and closure; note restoration of the contour of the plantar heel. (*I*) An RSAF after inset and partial closure. The distal aspect of the incision was left open in order to monitor the flap. (*J*) The RSAF after complete healing. (*Courtesy of* S. Masadeh, DPM, Cincinnati, OH.)

Table 2
Summary of the results/complications systematic reviews of the reverse sural artery flap

	No. of Patients (Flaps)	Percent Reported Smokers	Percent Reported with Diabetes Mellitus	Percent Reported with Peripheral Vascular Disease	Total Complications	Partial Flap Loss/ Necrosis	Total Flap Loss
Follmar et al,[1] 2007	720	n/a	n/a	n/a	133 (18)	76 (10.6)	24 (3.3)
de Blacam et al,[43] 2014	907	35	178	62	229 (26.4)	139 (15.3)	29 (3.2)
Daar et al,[44] 2020	479 (481)	34.6	35.4	12.3	128 (26.6)	74 (15.4)	15 (3.1)

Data are presented as N (%) unless otherwise specified.
Abbreviation: n/a, not applicable.
Data from Refs.[1,43,44]

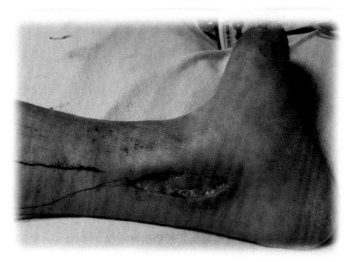

Fig. 27. Wound dehiscence with exposed vein graft after distal posterior tibial artery bypass graft for a patient with peripheral arterial disease. (*Courtesy of* S. Masadeh, DPM, Cincinnati, OH.)

- The RSAF is versatile and pliable, allowing for greater reach.
- The most common complication of the RSAF is partial flap necrosis owing to venous congestion.
- The RSAF has a higher rate of complications in patients with diabetes mellitus, peripheral vascular disease, and tobacco use.

DISCLOSURE

The authors have nothing to disclose.

REFERENCES

1. Follmar KE, Baccarani A, Baumeister SP, et al. The distally based sural flap. Plast Reconstr Surg 2007;119(6):138–48.
2. Masquelet AC, Romana MC, Wolf G. Skin island flaps Invited Discussion: Hallock: reverse sural artery flap supplied by the vascular axis of the sensitive superficial nerves: anatomic study and clinical experience in the leg. Plast Reconstr Surg 1992;89:1115–21.
3. Donski PK, Fogdestam I. Distally based fasciocutaneous flap from the sural region: a preliminary report. Scand J Plast Reconstr Surg 1983;17:191.
4. Basu A. Classification of flaps and application of the concept of vascular territories. 2016: 93–120.
5. Erovic BM, Lercher P. Classification of, . flaps. Manual of reconstruction using regional and free flaps. Vienna (Austria): Springer; 2015.
6. Taylor GI. The angiosomes of the body and their supply to perforator flaps. Clin Plast Surg 2003;30:330–41.
7. Schaverien M, Saint-Cyr M. Perforators of the lower leg: analysis of perforator locations and clinical application for pedicled perforator flaps. Plast Reconstr Surg 2008;122:160–70.

8. Yang D, Steven FM. Reversed sural island flap supplied by the lower septocutaneous perforator of the peroneal artery. Ann Plast Surg 2002;49(4):375–8.
9. Punyavong P, Winaikosol K, Jenwitheesuk K, et al. An anatomical study of vascular supply of the distally based sural artery flap: a cadaveric study. J Med Assoc Thai 2016;99(5):182–6.
10. Lee HI, Ha SH, Sun OY, et al. Reverse sural artery island flap with skin extension along the pedicle. J Foot Ankle Surg 2016;55(3):470–5.
11. Ward KL. Cadaveric atlas for orthoplastic lower limb and foot reconstruction of soft tissue defects. Clinics in Surgery 2018;3.
12. Imanishi N, Nakajima H, Fukuzumi S, et al. Venous drainage of the distally based lesser saphenous-sural veno-neuroadipofascial pedicled fasciocutaneous flap: a radiographic perfusion study. Plast Reconstr Surg 1999;103:494.
13. Price MF, Capizzi PJ, Watterson PA, et al. Reverse sural artery flap: caveats for success. Ann Plast Surg 2002;48(5):496–504.
14. Al-Quattan MM. A modified technique for harvesting the reverse sural artery flap from the upper part of the leg: inclusion of a gastrocnemius muscle "cuff" around the sural pedicle. Ann Plast Surg 2001;47:269.
15. Al-Quattan MM. Lower-limb reconstruction utilizing the reverse sural artery flap-gastrocnemius muscle cuff technique. Ann Plast Surg 2005;55:174.
16. Mahakkanukrauh P, Chomsung R. Anatomical variations of the sural nerve. Clin Anat 2002;15:263.
17. Ugrenovic S, Vasovic L, Jovanovic I, et al. Peculiarities of the sural nerve complex morphologic types in human fetuses. Surg Radiol Anat 2005;27:25.
18. Ortigiiela ME, Michael BW, Donald RC. Anatomy of the sural nerve complex. J Hand Surg 1987;12(6):1119–23.
19. Coert JH, Dellon AL. Clinical implications of the surgical anatomy of the sural nerve. Plast Reconstr Surg 1994;94(6):850–5.
20. Riedl O, Manfred F. Anatomy of the sural nerve: cadaver study and literature review. Plast Reconstr Surg 2013;131(4):802–10.
21. Kim H, Hu J, Chang H, et al. Sural nerve splitting in reverse sural artery perforator flap: anatomical study in 40 cadaver legs. Plast Reconstr Surg 2017;140(5):1024–32.
22. Tan O, Atik B, Bekerecioglu M. Supercharged reverse-flow sural flap: a new modification increasing the reliability of the flap. Microsurgery 2005;25:36.
23. Baumeister SP, Spierer R, Erdmann D, et al. A realistic complication analysis of 70 sural artery flaps in a multimorbid patient group. Plast Reconstr Surg 2003;112(1):129–40.
24. de Rezende MR, Saito M, Paulos RG, et al. Reduction of morbidity with a reverse-flow sural flap: a two-stage technique. J Foot Ankle Surg 2018;57(4):821–5.
25. Sugg KB, Schaub TA, Concannon MJ, et al. The reverse superficial sural artery flap revisited for complex lower extremity and foot reconstruction. Plast Reconstr Surg Glob Open 2015;3(9):e519.
26. Chang SM, Zhang K, Li HF, et al. Distally based sural fasciomyocutaneous flap: anatomic study and modified technique for complicated wounds of the lower third leg and weight bearing heel. Microsurgery 2009;9(23):205–13.
27. Zhang F, Lin S, Song Y, et al. Distally based sural neuro-lesser saphenous veno-fasciocutaneous compound flap with a low rotation point: microdissection and clinical application. Ann Plast Surg 2009;4(62):395–404.
28. Erdmann D, Gottlieb N, Humphrey JS, et al. Sural flap delay procedure: a preliminary report. Ann Plast Surg 2005;54:562.

29. Erdmann D, Levin S. Delayed reverse sural flap for staged reconstruction of the foot and lower leg. Plast Reconstr Surg 2006;118(2):571–2.
30. Kneser U, Bach AD, Polykandriotis E, et al. Delayed reverse sural flap for staged reconstruction of the foot and lower leg. Plast Reconstr Surg 2005; 116:1910.
31. Tosun Z, Ozkan A, Karacor Z, et al. Delaying the reverse sural flap provides predictable results for complicated wounds in diabetic foot. Ann Plast Surg 2005; 55:169.
32. Karacalar A, Idil O, Demir A, et al. Delay in neurovenous flaps: experimental and clinical experience. Ann Plast Surg 2004;53:481.
33. Angelats J, Albert LT. Sural nerve neurocutaneous cross-foot flap. Ann Plast Surg 1984;13:239.
34. Rajendra Prasad JS, Chaudhari C, Cunha-Gomes D, et al. The venoneuroadipo-fascial pedicled distally based sural island myofasciocutaneous flap: case reports. Br J Plast Surg 2002;55:210.
35. Ijpma FA, Jean-Phillipe A, Nicolai M, et al. Sural nerve donor-site morbidity: thirty-four years of follow-up. Ann Plast Surg 2006;57(4):391–5.
36. Hyakusoku H, Tonegawa H, Fumiiri M. Heel coverage with a T-shaped distally based sural island fasciocutaneous flap. Plast Reconstr Surg 1994; 93:872–6.
37. Aoki S, Tanuma K, Iwakiri I, et al. Clinical and vascular anatomical study of distally based sural flap. Ann Plast Surg 2008;1(61):73–8.
38. Aydin OE, Tan O, Kuduban SD, et al. Nerve sparing-distally based sural flap. Microsurgery 2011;4(31):276–80.
39. Le B, Fourn NC, Pannier M. Distally based sural fasciomuscular flap: anatomic study and application for filling leg or foot defects. Plast Reconstr Surg 2001; 107(1):67–72.
40. Bocchi A, Merelli S, Morellini A, et al. Reverse fasciosubcutaneous flap versus distally pedicled sural island flap: two elective methods for distal-third leg reconstruction. Ann Plast Surg 2000;45(3):284–91.
41. Chen S, Chen T, Chuo T, et al. Distally based sural fasciomusculocutaneous flap for chronic calcaneal osteomyelitis in diabetic patients. Ann Plast Surg 2005; 54:44.
42. Mueller JE, Ilchmann T, Lowatascheff T. The musculocutaneous sural artery flap for soft-tissue coverage after calcaneal fracture. Arch Orthop Trauma Surg 2001; 121:350.
43. de Blacam C, Colakoglu S, Ogunleye AA, et al. Risk factors associated with complications in lower-extremity reconstruction with the distally based sural flap: a systematic review and pooled analysis. J Plast Reconstr Aesthet Surg 2014; 67(5):607–16.
44. Daar DA, Abdou SA, David JA, et al. Revisiting the reverse sural artery flap in distal lower extremity reconstruction: a systematic review and risk analysis. Ann Plast Surg 2020;84(4):463–70.
45. Mohammadkhah N, Motamed S, Hosseini SN, et al. Complex technique of large sural flap: an alternative option for free flap in large defect of the traumatized foot. Acta Med Iran 2011;49:195–200.
46. Bibbo C. A modified anterior approach to the ankle. J Foot Ankle Surg 2013; 52(1):136–7.
47. Ducic I, Attinger CE. Foot and ankle reconstruction: pedicled muscle flaps versus free flaps and the role of diabetes. Plast Reconstr Surg 2011;128:173–80.

48. Jeng SF, Wei FC. Distally based sural island flap for foot and ankle reconstruction. Plast Reconstr Surg 1997;99:744–50.

49. Tsai J, Liao HT, Wang PF, et al. Increasing the success of reverse sural flap from proximal part of posterior calf for traumatic foot and ankle reconstruction: patient selection and surgical refinement. Microsurgery 2013;33(5):342–9.

50. Hong JP, Neligan PC, Song DH. Reconstructive surgery: lower extremity coverage. Reconstructive Surgery. 3rd edition. Philadelphia; 2013. p. 127-50.

51. Eser C, Kesiktaş E, Gencel E, et al. An alternative method to free flap for distal leg and foot defects due to electrical burn injury: distally based cross-leg sural flap. Ulus Travma Acil Cerrahi Derg 2016;1(22):46–51.

52. Hasegawa M, Torii S, Katoh H, et al. The distally based superficial sural artery flap. Plast Reconstr Surg 1994;5(93):1012–20.

Propeller Flaps of the Lower Extremity

Michael D. Liette, DPM[a], Pedro Rodriguez, MD[b], Christopher Bibbo, DO, DPM[c], Suhail Masadeh, DPM[d,*], Mohamed A. Ellabban, MD, MBBCh, MSc, MRCS[e]

KEYWORDS

- Propeller flap • Ulceration • Fasciocutaneous • Lower limb reconstruction
- Limb salvage • Perforator

KEY POINTS

- Lower extremity wounds involving the distal third of the leg are challenging to treat due to an often fragile soft tissue envelope, trauma, infection, hydrostatic pressures, edema, venous insufficiency, and peripheral vascular disease.
- Propeller flaps may provide coverage of these lower extremity wounds with manageable donor site morbidity.
- Adequate vascularity must be established prior to any surgical intervention. Acoustic or color Doppler may be sufficient to establish a perforator to base a propeller flap. Angiography and CT angiography also may be used.
- Design of the flap must minimize tension during inset to prevent kinking of the pedicle and minimize potential postoperative complications.
- Complications experienced often are minor in nature and readily managed conservatively.

INTRODUCTION

Wounds of the lower extremity, especially those of the distal third of the leg, pose significant challenges due to the unique anatomy and physiology of this region. The thin subcutaneous layer, multitude of superficial tendons, and lack of muscle over the anterior-medial-lateral limb regions contribute to the difficulty of wound management. Free flaps often are the procedure of choice in cases of immediate coverage needed. Patients with lower extremity wounds, however, often are frail and medically

[a] University of Cincinnati Medical Center, 231 Albert Sabin Way, ML 0513, Cincinnati, OH 45276, USA; [b] Plastic and Reconstructive Surgery, OSF Saint Anthony Medical Center, 698 Featherstone Road. Rockford, IL 61107, USA; [c] Foot and Ankle Surgery, Reconstructive Plastic and Microsurgery, and Limb Salvage, Musculoskeletal Infection and Orthopaedic Trauma, Rubin Institute for Advanced Orthopedics, International Center for Limb Lengthening, Sinai Hospital of Baltimore, 2401 West Belvedere Avenue, Baltimore, MD 21215-5216, USA; [d] University of Cincinnati Medical Center, Cincinnati Veteran Affairs Medical Center, 231 Albert Sabin Way, ML 0513, Cincinnati, OH 45276, USA; [e] Suez Canal University Hospitals and Medical School, Ismailia 41522, Egypt
* Corresponding author.
E-mail address: masadesb@uc.edu

Clin Podiatr Med Surg 37 (2020) 727–742
https://doi.org/10.1016/j.cpm.2020.06.001
0891-8422/20/Published by Elsevier Inc.

compromised, with suboptimal physiology to rise to the threshold needed to experience these time-consuming procedures. Furthermore, free tissue transfers require highly specialized skills and a medical facility able to support microsurgery demands. The knowledge of soft tissue perfusion has evolved rapidly, allowing the use of fasciocutaneous rotation flaps to assume a larger role in the reconstructive algorithm. Fasciocutaneous rotation flaps, including the propeller-style flap, have proved reliable, relatively quick, often capable of providing a more aesthetically pleasing outcome, and to have significantly less host morbidity without disturbing the axial source vessels or the intracompartmental muscles.[1-3]

ANATOMY OF A PERFORATOR-BASED PROPELLER FLAP

The Tokyo consensus defined a propeller flap as an island fasciocutaneous flap that is axially rotated between 90° and 180° on an established perforator, or pedicle, to cover a local soft tissue deficit.[4] Perforators have been defined as the blood vessels that branch from an axial source vessel and travel onward to the subcutaneous fat region, or subdermal plexus, either directly through the septum or through the muscle; this concept is visualized in **Fig. 1**.[5] The tissues through which the perforator travels to reach the subdermal plexus define the type of perforator and may be classified as direct cutaneous, septocutaneous, or musculocutaneous.[5-7] The propeller flap requires a thorough understanding of the perforasome concept to ensure appropriate preoperative planning and adequate postoperative outcomes are achieved. This is the cutaneous territory, or domain, supplied by a single perforator through both the direct and indirect connections between adjacent perforators within the subdermal plexus.[8] The direct connections occur via larger linking vessels, capable of connecting multiple perforasomes together through direct anastomoses.[8] The indirect connections occur via the dense arboreal anastomotic network within the subdermal plexus, as seen in **Fig. 2**.[8] These connections between perforators allow for large propeller flaps to be raised and rotated around a single perforator, with reliable perfusion

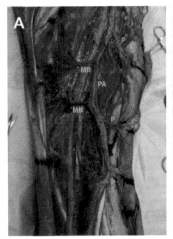
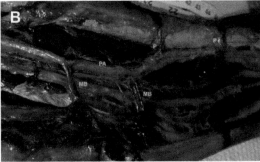

Fig. 1. (*A, B*) Visualized is the peroneal artery (PA) and multiple septocutaneous perforators with accompanying venae comitantes (P) as well as several muscular branches (MB) within the lateral compartment of the leg. (*Courtesy of* S. Masadeh, DPM, Cincinnati, OH.)

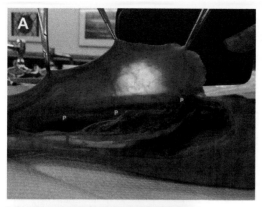

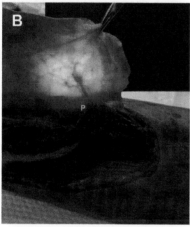

Fig. 2. (*A, B*) Visualized are the perforators (P) based on the peroneal artery and the dense arboreal anastomotic network within the subdermal plexus providing indirect connections between adjacent perforasomes. (*Courtesy of* S. Masadeh, DPM, Cincinnati, OH.)

throughout the entirety of the flap through both direct and retrograde flow throughout adjacent perforasomes.

The 3 main axial source vessels of the lower extremity—the posterior tibial artery, the peroneal artery, and the anterior tibial artery—have well-established perforators with reliable anatomic locations. These perforators may be harvested individually, along with their accompanying fasciocutaneous domains, and rotated to cover various lower extremity wounds. A cadaveric study performed by Schaverien and Saint-Cyr[9] evaluated the anatomic location of these perforators and found them to be located within the intermuscular septum at approximately 5-cm intervals from the level of the malleoli; this is visualized in **Fig. 3**. These intervals, beginning distally at the malleoli and traveling proximal, ranged from 4 cm to 9 cm to 13 cm to 18 cm to 21 cm to 26 cm.[9] The peroneal artery–based propeller flaps may provide soft tissue coverage for deficits overlying the lateral malleolus or the Achilles tendon; an example is seen in **Fig. 4**.[2,10,11] The posterior tibial artery–based flaps may provide coverage of anterior tibial, medial malleolar, or Achilles tendon deficits.[9,10,12,13] The tibialis anterior flaps often are used for the coverage of deficits of the anterior tibia, medial and lateral malleoli, or anterior ankle deficits.[10,14,15] Determining which axial source vessel to base a

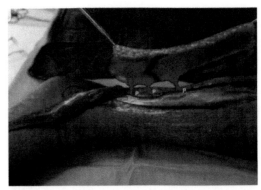

Fig. 3. Multiple perforators (P) upon which propeller flap may be based for rotation pending on further clinical examination. Chosen perforator is identified based on vascular perfusion and length required for rotation. (*Courtesy of* S. Masadeh, DPM, Cincinnati, OH.)

perforator off of is determined by the anatomic location of the soft tissue defect requiring coverage and a vascular examination.

CLINICAL APPLICATIONS AND SURGICAL TECHNIQUE

The design of the propeller flap begins with a thorough vascular examination utilizing either acoustic or color Doppler of both the axial vessel and the associated perforators to ensure adequate vascularity is present. Acoustic Doppler examination provides a rapid, reproducible means to evaluate both the location and the relative vascular supply of the perforators through the phasic activity of the vessel and the loudness of the examination.[1,16–18] Color Doppler is capable of providing greater detail of the vasculature and allows for visualization of the internal diameter and the velocity of flow within

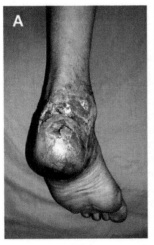
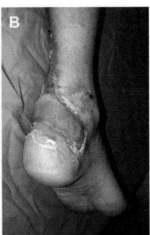
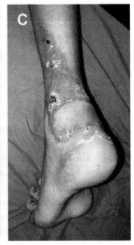

Fig. 4. (*A–C*) Visualized is a traumatic induced posterior Achilles deficit treated with a peroneal artery–based propeller flap. Harvest site was primarily closed and flap was rotated to final inset position, maintaining the physiologic soft tissue contour of the region. (*Courtesy of* S. Masadeh, DPM, Cincinnati, OH.)

the perforators; this is visualized in **Fig. 5**. This test has been shown to be reliable in determining the perforator with the largest vascularized territory based on the internal diameter, the velocity, and the perfusion pressure measurements.[2,19,20] Bhattacharya and colleagues[19] showed that a larger diameter perforator had increased velocity and higher perfusion pressure, and therefore a larger cutaneous domain, or perforasome. Utilizing a Doppler examination preoperatively avoids the use of an exploratory incision and the risks associated with this to accurately identify the perforator locations. This simple exam significantly improves the reliability of propeller flaps because intraoperative dissection of a perforator is technically demanding. Preoperative identification of the locations reduces the chance of complications or damage to the perforators and ensures harvest of the correct vessel. If Doppler examination proves unreliable, several investigators have advocated the use of preoperative angioscanning or computed tomography angiography to evaluate the perforators in even greater detail to aid in preoperative flap design.[21]

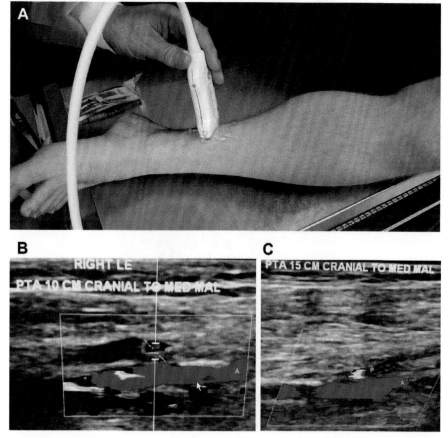

Fig. 5. (*A–C*) Visualized is the use of color Doppler examination to identify the locations of perforating arteries (P) along their dominant source artery (A). These can be identified and marked preoperatively to provide more information about flap design and viability. (*Courtesy of* S. Masadeh, DPM, Cincinnati, OH.)

After Doppler examination is complete and the perforator to be harvested has been identified, the propeller flap may be further designed based on the location and the size of the soft tissue deficit. The flap ideally is based on the perforator closest to the deficit to avoid the need for the creation of a longer skin island and an increased potential of distal flap necrosis, but a thorough vascular examination always must be performed prior to selection. A flap with a larger cutaneous area is reliant on the perfusion of multiple adjacent perforasomes through the indirect connections within the subdermal plexus and may be more prone to necrosis at the distal aspect, which often is the critical portion most needed for deficit coverage. When designing the flap preoperatively, the margins should exceed the margins of the soft tissue deficit to avoid excess tension and minimize complications after inset from soft tissue contracture.[22] To outline the dimensions of the flap, the distance from the perforator to the distal edge of the deficit is measured and 1 cm is added to this to minimize the tension.[22] This measurement is the length of the fasciocutaneous flap necessary to harvest extending from the pedicle proximally, to allow for rotation and coverage of the deficit;

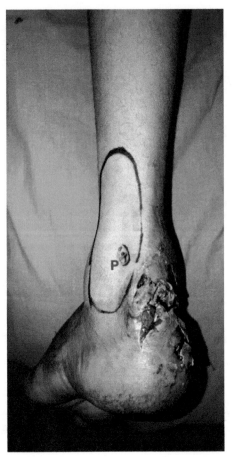

Fig. 6. Flap is designed after Doppler examination to identify the perforator upon which the flap will be based (P). The margins then are outlined so that the flap will fill the soft tissue deficit with excess margins to ensure minimal tension is placed during final inset. (*Courtesy of* S. Masadeh, DPM, Cincinnati, OH.)

this is demonstrated in **Fig. 6**. The width of the deficit to be filled is measured next, and 0.5 cm is added to this measurement to additionally ensure tension is at a minimum during the inset.[22]

After identification of the perforator to be harvested and the design of the propeller flap is complete, elevation of the flap may begin. Dissection may be carried out either suprafascial or subfascial to identify the perforators, because this has been shown in a systematic review and meta-analysis performed by Bekara and colleagues[1] to have no significant difference in complications or postoperative course. Once identification of the selected perforator is complete, further dissection may be carried out to free the perforator and venae comitantes from the surroundings septum and soft tissue attachments, otherwise known as skeletonizing the pedicle; this is visualized in **Fig. 7**.[1,23–26] Skeletonizing the pedicle allows for maximal of the pedicle length, minimizes flow resistance and endothelial damage, and produces minimal tension on the pedicle and venae comitantes, thereby maximizing the perfusion pressures and the area of vascularized tissue capable of being harvested.[1,23–26] Wong and colleagues[27] demonstrated that a perforator with a pedicle length of at least 3 cm and a diameter of 1 mm has a significantly decreased risk of kinking during rotation from increased torsion. Regardless of the pedicle length achieved, Demir and colleagues[28] showed that

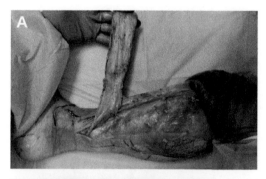

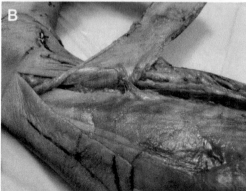

Fig. 7. (*A*) Demonstrates the elevation of posterior tibial artery–based propeller flap for medial ankle soft tissue coverage. Demonstrated is the pedicle within the septum and the fasciocutaneous margins of the flap. (*B*) Visualized is the perforator with accompanying venae comitantes upon which flap is propelled to final inset position. The surrounding soft tissues are skeletonized to allow for fully uninhibited rotation around the perforator. (*Courtesy of* S. Masadeh, DPM, Cincinnati, OH.)

serious compromise of perforator integrity is seen with axial rotations greater than 180° and the likelihood of pursuant flap necrosis is increased significantly. Therefore, flap rotation should be in the direction of the smaller arc of rotation to maximize perfusion pressures and minimize complications.[28]

Prior to rotation, adequate perfusion must be established to the elevated island fasciocutaneous flap, ensuring that a vasospasm of the pedicle has not occurred after ligation of the surrounding perforators. It is a critical step to wait 15 minutes to 20 minutes to allow for any potential choke vessels to open in-between the perforasomes through the opening of the direct and indirect communications to allow for better perfusion of the flap.[24,25] This process may be encouraged with the use of vasodilators, such as lidocaine, papaverine, or warmed saline placed, around the pedicle to alleviate a vasospasm as well as promote the dilation of additional vascular channels within the flap margins.[24,25] In the circumstance that the flap experiences vasospasm after initial rotation, it advisable to again use vasodilators to alleviate the spasm. Should the vasospasm continue to persist, it is recommended to return the flap to the donor site and delay the procedure until improved vascularity is achieved and additional vascular channels are opened to assist perfusion during a later rotation, as seen in **Fig. 8**.[24,25]

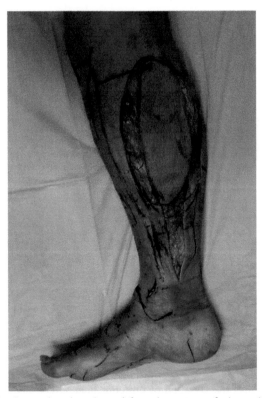

Fig. 8. Flap is fully elevated and evaluated for adequate perfusion prior to rotation and inset. This may be performed through Doppler examination, capillary refill time, and bleeding edges. Should the flap show signs of inadequate perfusion, it is returned to harvest site and the procedure is delayed, allowing for further vascularization to develop. (*Courtesy of* S. Masadeh, DPM, Cincinnati, OH.)

Table 1
Peroneal artery perforator propeller flap results

	Number of Propeller Flaps	Propeller Elevation	Complications	Partial Flap Necrosis	Total Flap Necrosis	Average Follow-up
Koshima et al,[29] 2003	9	—	2	2	0	—
Jakubietz et al,[2] 2007	5	Suprafascial	1	1	0	6 mo
Mun et al,[30] 2008	1	Suprafascial	0	0	0	10 mo
Pignatti et al,[31] 2008	1	Subfascial	0	0	0	—
Rad et al,[11] 2008	1	—	0	0	0	24 mo
Sananpanich et al,[32] 2008	21	—	3	2	1	—
Bhat et al,[33] 2009	1	Subfascial	0	0	0	8 mo
Rubino et al,[34] 2009	1	Subfascial	0	0	0	12 mo
Jakubietz et al,[35] 2010	3	Subfascial	0	0	0	—
Lecours et al,[36] 2010	4	Subfascial	1	1	0	—
Rezende et al,[37] 2010	9	Subfascial	0	0	0	—
D'Arpa et al,[24] 2011	4	Subfascial	1	1	0	—
Higueras Suñé et al,[21] 2011	7	Subfascial	3	3	0	—
Lu et al,[38] 2011	11	Subfascial	4	1	0	—
Ono et al,[39] 2011	2	—	0	0	0	—
Tos et al,[40] 2011	6	Subfascial	4	2	0	6 mo
Karki and Narayan,[41] 2012	6	Subfascial	1	1	0	13.2 mo
Mateev and Kuokkanen,[42] 2012	4	—	0	0	0	—
Shin et al,[43] 2012	3	Subfascial	2	1	1	7.7 mo
Totals	99	—	22 (22%)	15 (15%)	2 (2%)	6–24 mo

Data from Refs.[2,11,21,24,29–43]

Table 2
Posterior tibial artery perforator propeller flap results

	Number of Propeller Flaps	Propeller Elevation	Complications	Partial Necrosis/ Epidermal Necrosis	Full Necrosis	Follow-up
Kohsima et al,[29] 2003	1	—	0	0	0	17 mo
Koshima et al,[13] 2005	1	—	0	0	0	—
Jakubietz et al,[2] 2007	3	Suprafascial	2	2	0	6 mo
Mun et al,[30] 2008	1	Suprafascial	0	0	0	10 mo
Pignatti et al,[31] 2008	1	Subfascial	1	1	0	—
Sananpanich et al,[32] 2008	4	—	1	0	0	—
Bhat et al,[33] 2009	5	Subfascial	2	2	0	8 mo
Bravo and Schwarze,[23] 2009	2	Subfascial	1	0	0	8.5 mo
Bous et al,[44] 2011	2	Subfascial	0	0	0	12 mo
Jakubietz et al,[35] 2010	2	Subfascial	2	1	1	—
Lecours et al,[36] 2010	10	Subfascial	3	1	1	—
Rezende et al,[37] 2010	10	Subfascial	1	1	0	—
Robotti et al,[45] 2010	24	Subfascial	3	2	0	13 mo
Schaverien et al,[46] 2010	106	Subfascial	34	12	9	6 mo
D'Arpa et al,[24] 2011	7	Subfascial	2	1	0	—
Higueras Suñé et al,[21] 2011	1	Subfascial	0	0	0	—
Ignatiadis et al,[47] 2011	5	—	2	1	0	18–84 mo
Ono et al,[39] 2011	3	—	0	0	0	—
Tos et al,[40] 2011	13	Subfascial	4	4	0	6 mo
Karki and Narayan,[41] 2012	14	Subfascial	3	0	0	10.2 mo
Mateev and Kuokkanen,[42] 2012	4	—	2	0	1	—
Shin et al,[43] 2012	5	Subfascial	1	1	0	5 mo
Sharma et al,[48] 2012	10	Suprafascial	2	1	1	6 mo
Totals	234	—	66 (28%)	30 (13%)	13 (5.6%)	6–17 mo

Table 3
Anterior tibial artery perforator propeller flap results

	Number of Propeller Flaps	Propeller Elevation	Complications	Partial Necrosis/ Epidermal Necrosis	Full Necrosis	Average Follow-up
Mun et al,[30] 2008	1	Suprafascial	0	0	0	10 mo
Pignatti et al,[31] 2008	1	Subfascial	0	0	0	—
Lecours et al,[36] 2010	2	Subfascial	1	0	0	—
Rad et al,[15] 2010	4	Subfascial	2	1	0	12 mo
Rezende et al,[37] 2010	5	Subfascial	3	3	0	—
Totals	13	—	6 (46%)	4 (31%)	0 (0%)	10–12 mo

Data from Refs.[15,30,31,36,37]

RESULTS

Several studies have evaluated the use of perforator-based propeller flaps for the management of various soft tissue deficits of the lower extremity. The peroneal artery, posterior tibial artery, and the anterior tibial artery–based perforator propeller flaps were isolated within these studies for review. Soft tissue deficits evaluated within these studies were noted to occur from a variety of etiologies, including trauma, ulceration, burns, scars, vascular disease, infection, and malignancy. The results of these studies are summarized in **Tables 1–3**.[1,2,11,13,15,21,23,24,29–48]

DISCUSSION

Wounds of the lower extremity often are difficult to manage due to the poor soft tissue envelope of the lower leg, with vital structures often located superficially beneath the skin surface. The lower extremity has additional unique challenges for coverage options because the soft tissue envelope in this area is very thin with less of a subcutaneous compartment compared with other regions of the body, the superficial location of the tendons, and a lack of musculature capable of providing the necessary vascularized wound beds for healing. These wounds pose significant morbidity and mortality to patients and have the potential to lead to infection or progress onward to amputation if not managed properly at the initial presentation. The use of local perforator-based fasciocutaneous propeller flaps has proved an excellent option to provide rapid coverage of lower extremity deficits while maintaining minimal host morbidity. They are capable of minimizing the duration of an open wound and preventing the development of deep infection by providing rapid vascularized soft tissue coverage. Because the donor site often is able to be primarily closed or immediately skin grafted, due to the presence of underlying intracompartmental muscles and the maintenance of a vascularized wound bed during harvest, propellers may provide the additional benefits of providing an ideal cosmetic outcome by replacing the deficit with similar tissue that was lost.

Perforator-based propeller flaps have been evaluated by several investigators with great overall flap success and variable rates of complications. The studies isolated for review were limited to the selected propeller flaps of the lower extremity and demonstrated excellent overall results in their use for the management of soft tissue deficits of the lower extremity, with few absolute failures noted. The studies evaluating the peroneal artery perforator–based propeller flap experienced a complication rate of approximately 22%, with a majority of these complications minor and including venous congestion, superficial partial necrosis, and epidermolysis.[2,11,21,24,29–43] The rate of complete flap failure with total necrosis was found approximately 2%.[2,11,21,24,29–43] The studies evaluating the posterior tibial artery perforator–based propeller flaps were significantly larger in comparison than those for the other 2 propeller flaps evaluated in this review. They found the rate of complete flap necrosis to be approximately 5.6%, and an overall complication rate of approximately 28%, of which the main complications appeared again to be minor in nature and included venous congestion, superficial partial necrosis, and epidermolysis.[2,13,21,23,24,29–33,35–37,39–48] The anterior tibial artery–based perforator propeller flaps, with only 13 flaps evaluated, demonstrated an overall complication rate of approximately 46%, with none of these going on to complete necrosis or failure.[15,30,31,36,37] A vast majority of complications noted were minor, often readily managed conservatively without significant morbidity to the patient. The overall rate of flap failure was found quite low within these isolated studies, with approximately 4.3% of flaps experiencing total necrosis after rotation and inset.[1,2,11,13,15,21,23,24,29–48]

A recent systematic review, a meta-analysis performed by Bekar and colleagues,[1] showed similar rates of complications and failures as seen within this review. The investigators found rates of complete flap survival of various propellers of 84.3% and a rate of failure with total necrosis of 3.5%.[1] These findings were supported further in studies performed by Gir and colleagues[49] and Nelson and colleagues,[50] with comparable rates of total flap necrosis seen. Propeller flaps have shown slightly lower rates of total necrosis compared with their free flap counterparts, with rates of total free flap necrosis ranging from 4.1% to 5.9%.[51,52] Because free flaps have significantly more host morbidity, require extensive operating room time, are more technically demanding, and have the potential for a higher rate of complications and necrosis than local perforator-based propeller flaps, propellers appear to be an excellent first-choice option to manage wounds of the lower extremity, with free flaps reserved for secondary procedures should the propeller fail.[1,53,54]

When major complications occur, they often are related to partial flap necrosis, total necrosis, dehiscence, arterial insufficiency, venous congestion, or venous obstruction, leading to eventual flap failure. These may occur with higher rates in those patients with an age greater than 60, diabetes, or peripheral vascular disease.[1] Complications, if managed appropriately when first discovered, often are successful in salvaging the flap and avoiding return trips to the operating room for revision procedures. In the review performed by Bekar and colleagues,[1] they found rates of complications requiring a return to the operating room for revision in only 2.99% of cases. Overall, minor complications were seen in 6.5% of the cases, with superficial partial flap necrosis the most common complication, at a rate of 10.2%.[1] The partial necrosis likely was due to venous congestion within the flap, with rates of congestion seen in 3.5% after rotation and inset of the flap.[1] Because veins have a lower pressure system and, therefore, are more likely to kink during rotation, producing poor outflow capabilities; this is the more likely complication to occur rather than arterial insufficiency after inset.[1] This often may be managed conservatively by reducing tension on the flap and improving venous outflow with removal of the stitches, leech therapy, or, as recent studies performed by Qiu and colleagues[55] have shown, early application of negative pressure wound therapy.[4] If conservative measures are ineffective in alleviating the congestion, return to the operating room must be considered for re-evaluation of the flap inset and the potential for delay of the flap to allow for additional vascular channels prior to rotation or supercharging of the flap with a venous anastomosis to improve outflow capabilities or to alleviate any venous obstruction.[4,36]

Perforator-based propeller flaps require a significant understanding of the vascular anatomy of the lower extremity as well as training in microdissection techniques. They are capable of providing a reliable means of covering lower extremity soft tissues deficits while maintaining minimal morbidity to the host compared with free flaps. They provide the additional advantage over random pattern pedicle flaps, such as bilobed or trilobed flaps, because they ensure the incorporation of a perforator and its' vascular supply of the harvested perforasome, improving the chances of successful wound coverage. The results of these studies provide further evidence for the reliability of these flaps in the coverage of small to medium sized defects of the lower extremity with relatively low rates of overall complications and failures experienced after inset.

CLINICAL CARE POINTS

- Lower extremity wounds involving the distal third of the leg are challenging to treat due to an often fragile soft tissue envelope, trauma, infection, hydrostatic pressures, edema, venous insufficiency, and peripheral vascular disease.

- Propeller flaps may provide coverage of these lower extremity wounds with manageable donor site morbidity.
- Adequate vascularity must be established prior to any surgical intervention. Acoustic or color Doppler may be sufficient to establish a perforator to base a propeller flap. Angiography and CT angiography also may be used.
- Design of the flap must minimize tension during inset to prevent kinking of the pedicle and minimize potential postoperative complications.
- Complications experienced often are minor in nature and readily managed conservatively.
- Failure rates of perforator-based propeller flaps are similar to that of lower extremity soft tissue free flaps.

DISCLOSURE

The authors have nothing to disclose.

REFERENCES

1. Bekara F, Herlin C, Mojallal A, et al. A systematic review and meta-analysis of perforator-pedicled propeller flaps in lower extremity defects. Plast Reconstr Surg 2016;137(1):314–31.
2. Jakubietz RG, Jakubietz MG, Gruenert JG, et al. The 180-degree perforator-based propeller flap for soft tissue coverage of the distal, lower extremity: a new method to achieve reliable coverage of the distal lower extremity with a local, fasciocutaneous perforator flap. Ann Plast Surg 2007;59(6):667–71.
3. Song S, Jeong HH, Lee Y, et al. Direction of flap rotation in propeller flaps: does it really matter? J Reconstr Microsurg 2019;35:549–56.
4. Pignatti M, Ogawa R, Hallock GG, et al. The "Tokyo" consensus on propeller flaps. Plast Reconstr Surg 2011;127(2):716–22.
5. Blondeel PN, Van Landuyt KHI, Monstrey SJM, et al. The "Gent" consensus on perforator flap terminology: Preliminary definitions. Plast Reconstr Surg 2003;112(5):1378–82.
6. Hallock GG. Direct and indirect perforator flaps: the history and the controversy. Plast Reconstr Surg 2003;111(2):855–65.
7. Wei FC, Jain V, Suominen S, et al. Confusion among perforator flaps: what is a true perforator flap? Plast Reconstr Surg 2001;107(3):874–6.
8. Saint-Cyr M, Wong C, Schaverien M, et al. The perforasome theory: vascular anatomy and clinical implications. Plast Reconstr Surg 2009;124(5):1529–44.
9. Schaverien M, Saint-Cyr M. Perforators of the lower leg: analysis of perforator locations and clinical application for pedicled perforator flaps. Plast Reconstr Surg 2008;122(1):161–70.
10. Parrett B, Talbot S, Pribaz J, et al. A review of local and regional flaps for distal leg reconstruction. J Reconstr Microsurg 2009;25(07):445–55.
11. Rad AN, Singh NK, Rosson GD. Peroneal artery perforator-based propeller flap reconstruction of the lateral distal lower extremity after tumor extirpation: case report and literature review. Microsurgery 2008;28(8):663–70.
12. Koshima I, Moriguchi T, Ohta S, et al. The vasculature and clinical application of the posterior tibial perforator-based flap. Plast Reconstr Surg 1992;90(4):643–9.
13. Koshima I, Ozaki T, Gonda K, et al. Posterior tibial adiposal flap for repair of wide, full-thickness defect of the Achilles tendon. J Reconstr Microsurg 2005;21(8):551–4.

14. Kilinc H, Bilen BT, Arslan A. A novel flap to repair medial and lateral malleolar defects: anterior tibial artery perforator-based adipofascial flap. Ann Plast Surg 2006;57(4):396–401.
15. Rad AN, Christy MR, Rodriguez ED, et al. The anterior tibialis artery perforator (ATAP) flap for traumatic knee and patella defects: clinical cases and anatomic study. Ann Plast Surg 2010;64(2):210–6.
16. Blondeel PN, Beyens G, Verhaeghe R, et al. Doppler flowmetry in the planning of perforator flaps. Br J Plast Surg 1998;51(3):202–9.
17. Giunta RE, Geisweid A, Feller AM. The value of preoperative Doppler sonography for planning free perforator flaps. Plast Reconstr Surg 2000;105(7):2381–6.
18. Khan UD, Miller JG. Reliability of handheld Doppler in planning local perforator-based flaps for extremities. Aesthetic Plast Surg 2007;31(5):521–5.
19. Bhattacharya V, Deshpande SB, Watts RK, et al. Measurement of perfusion pressure of perforators and its correlation with their internal diameter. Br J Plast Surg 2005;58(6):759–64.
20. Geis S, Prantl L, Dolderer J, et al. Post- operative monitoring of local and free flaps with contrast- enhanced ultrasound (CEUS)–analysis of 112 patients. Ultraschall Med 2013;34(06):550–8.
21. Higueras Suñé MC, López Ojeda A, Narváez García JA, et al. Use of angioscanning in the surgical planning of perforator flaps in the lower extremities. J Plast Reconstr Aesthet Surg 2011;64:1207–13.
22. Teo TC. The propeller flap concept. Clin Plast Surg 2010;37(4):615–26.
23. Bravo FG, Schwarze HP. Free-style local perforator flaps: concept and classification system. J Plast Reconstr Aesthet Surg 2009;62(5):602–8.
24. D'Arpa S, Cordova A, Pignatti M, et al. Freestyle pedicled perforator flaps: safety, prevention of complications, and management based on 85 consecutive cases. Plast Reconstr Surg 2011;128(4):892–906.
25. D'Arpa S, Toia F, Pirrello R, et al. Propeller flaps: a review of indications, technique, and results. Biomed Res Int 2014;2014:1–7.
26. Selvaggi G, Anicic S, Formaggia L. Mathematical explanation of the buckling of the vessels after twisting of the microanastomosis. Microsurgery 2006;26(7):524–8.
27. Wong CH, Cui F, Tan BK, et al. Nonlinear finite element simulations to elucidate the determinants of perforator patency in propeller flaps. Ann Plast Surg 2007;59(6):672–8.
28. Demir A, Acar M, Yildix L, et al. The effect of twisting on perforator flap viability. An experimental study in rats. Ann Plast Surg 2006;56(2):186–9.
29. Koshima I, Itoh S, Nanba Y, et al. Medial and lateral malleolar perforator flaps for repair of defects around the ankle. Ann Plast Surg 2003;51:579–83.
30. Mun GH, Jo YW, Lim SY, et al. Pedicled perforator flap of stellate design. J Plast Reconstr Aesthet Surg 2008;61:1332–7.
31. Pignatti M, Pasqualini M, Governa M, et al. Propeller flaps for leg reconstruction. J Plast Reconstr Aesthet Surg 2008;61:777–83.
32. Sananpanich K, Tu YK, Kraisarin J, et al. Reconstruction of limb soft-tissue defects: using pedicle perforator flaps with preservation of major vessels, a report of 45 cases. Injury 2008;39(4):55–66.
33. Bhat S, Shah A, Burd A. The role of freestyle perforator- based pedicled flaps in reconstruction of delayed traumatic defects. Ann Plast Surg 2009;63:45–52.
34. Rubino C, Figus A, Mazzocchi M, et al. The propeller flap for chronic osteomyelitis of the lower extremities: a case report. J Plast Reconstr Aesthet Surg 2009;62:40–404.

35. Jakubietz RG, Jakubietz DF, Gruenert JG, et al. Reconstruction of soft tissue defects of the Achilles tendon with rotation flaps, pedicled propeller flaps and free perforator flaps. Microsurgery 2010;30:608–13.

36. Lecours C, Saint-Cyr M, Wong C, et al. Freestyle pedicle perforator flaps: clinical results and vascular anatomy. Plast Reconstr Surg 2010;126:1589–603.

37. Rezende MR, Rabelo NT, Wei TH, et al. Skin coverage of the middle-distal segment of the leg with a pedicled perforator flap. J Orthop Trauma 2010;24:236–43.

38. Lu TC, Lin CH, Lin CH, et al. Versatility of the pedicled peroneal artery perforator flaps for soft-tis- sue coverage of the lower leg and foot defects. J Plast Reconstr Aesthet Surg 2011;64:386–93.

39. Ono S, Chung KC, Hayashi H, et al. Application of multidetector-row computed tomography in propeller flap planning. Plast Reconstr Surg 2011;127:703–11.

40. Tos P, Innocenti M, Artiaco S, et al. Perforator-based propeller flaps treating loss of substance in the lower limb. J Orthop Traumatol 2011;12:93–9.

41. Karki D, Narayan RP. The versatility of perforator-based pro- peller flap for reconstruction of distal leg and ankle defects. Plast Surg Int 2012;2012:303247.

42. Mateev MA, Kuokkanen HO. Reconstruction of soft tissue defects in the extremities with a pedicled perforator flap: series of 25 patients. J Plast Surg Hand Surg 2012;46:32–6.

43. Shin IS, Lee DW, Rah DK, et al. Reconstruction of pre- tibial defect using pedicled perforator flaps. Arch Plast Surg 2012;39:360–6.

44. Bous A, Ronsmans C, Nizet JL, et al. The perforator pedicled propeller flap for distal tibial exposure: two case reports. Ann Chir Plast Esthet 2011;56:562–7.

45. Robotti E, Carminati M, Bonfirraro PP, et al. "On demand" posterior tibial artery perforator flaps: a versatile surgical procedure for reconstruction of soft tissue defects of the leg after tumor excision. Ann Plast Surg 2010;64:202–9.

46. Schaverien MV, Hamilton SA, Fairburn N, et al. Lower limb reconstruction using the islanded posterior tibial artery perforator flap. Plast Reconstr Surg 2010; 125:1735–43.

47. Ignatiadis IA, Georgakopoulos GD, Tsiampa VA, et al. Distal posterior tibial artery perforator flaps for the management of calcaneal and Achilles tendon injuries in diabetic and non-diabetic patients. Diabet Foot Ankle 2011;2. https://doi.org/10.3402/dfa.v2i0.7483.

48. Sharma M, Balasubramanian D, Thankappan K, et al. Propeller flaps in the closure of free fibula flap donor site skin defects. Ann Plast Surg 2013;71:76–9.

49. Gir P, Cheng A, Oni G, et al. Pedicled-perforator (propeller) flaps in lower extremity defects: a systematic review. J Reconstr Microsurg 2012;28(09):595–602.

50. Nelson JA, Fischer JP, Brazio PS, et al. A review of propeller flaps for distal lower extremity soft tissue reconstruction: is flap loss too high? Microsurgery 2013; 33(7):578–86.

51. Fischer JP, Wink JD, Nelson JA, et al. A retrospective review of outcomes and flap selection in free tissue transfers for complex lower extremity reconstruction. J Reconstr Microsurg 2013;29:407–16.

52. Wettstein R, Schürch R, Banic A, et al. Review of 197 consecutive free flap reconstructions in the lower extremity. J Plast Reconstr Aesthet Surg 2008;61:772–6.

53. Hiakusoku H, Ogawa R, Oky K, et al. The perforator pedicled propeller (PPP) flap method: report of two cases. J Nippon Med Sch 2007;74(5):367–71.

54. Geddes CR, Morris SF, Neligan PC. Perforator flaps: evolution, classification, and applications. Ann Plast Surg 2003;50(1):90–9.

55. Qiu SS, Hsu CC, Hanna SA, et al. Negative pressure wound therapy for the management of flaps with venous congestion. Microsugery 2016;36(6):467–73.

Local and Regional Flaps in Pedal Reconstruction (Muscle and Fasciocutaneous Flaps)

Understanding the Arterial Anatomy and Dermal Perfusion of the Lower Extremity with Clinical Application

Stephanie Oexeman, DPM, Kaitlyn L. Ward, DPM*

KEYWORDS

- Perforators • Lower extremity • Angiosomes • Arterial anatomy • Dermal perfusion

KEY POINTS

- Respecting vascular territories is crucial for flap design.
- Reliable perforators of the lower extremity are found in intervals.
- Various preoperative modalities can help identify perforators.

INTRODUCTION

An in-depth knowledge of the vasculature of the lower extremity is necessary for planning the most advantageous surgical procedures. Understanding these principles not only helps surgeons choose the correct procedures but also allows for optimal healing.[1,2]

ANGIOSOMES OF THE LOWER EXTREMITY

There are at least 40 angiosomes present throughout the body, including 6 within the foot and ankle originating from the 3 major arteries of the lower extremity: posterior tibial, anterior tibial, and peroneal arteries (**Fig. 1**). Each artery has distinct borders within the angiosome boundaries.[1,2]

The Posterior Tibial Artery

The posterior tibial artery is the powerhouse of the lower leg, supplying the superficial and deep compartment muscles. Continuing from the popliteal artery, the posterior tibial artery originates distal to the popliteal fossa and courses distally behind the

Complex Deformity Correction & Microsurgical Limb Reconstruction Fellowship, AMITA Health-St. Joseph Hospital, Attn: Podiatric Fellowship Office, 2900 North Lake Shore Drive, Chicago, IL 60657, USA
* Corresponding author.
E-mail address: Kaitlynlward@gmail.com

Clin Podiatr Med Surg 37 (2020) 743–749
https://doi.org/10.1016/j.cpm.2020.07.003
0891-8422/20/© 2020 Elsevier Inc. All rights reserved.

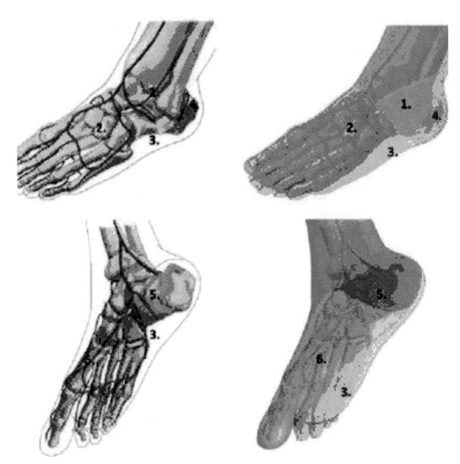

Fig. 1. The currently described foot angiosomes. (1) The anterior communicant angiosome (from the peroneal artery). (2) Dorsalis pedis angiosome (from the anterior tibial artery). (3) Lateral plantar angiosome (from the posterior tibial artery). (4) Lateral calcaneal angiosome (from the peroneal artery). (5) Medial calcaneal angiosome (from the posterior tibial artery). (6) Medial plantar angiosome (from the posterior tibial artery). (*From* Alexandrescu VA, Sinatra T, Maufroy C. Current Issues and Interrogations in Angiosome Wound Targeted Revascularization for Chronic Limb Threatening Ischemia: A Review. World J Cardiovasc Dis. 2019;9(3):168-192; with permission.)

tibialis posterior tendon. Within the upper third of the lower leg, the peroneal artery branches off.[1,2] As the posterior tibial artery travels distally toward the ankle, the artery can be located posterior to the medial malleolus supplying the medial ankle and eventually dividing into its 3 main branches: the medial plantar, the lateral plantar, and calcaneal arteries.[1,2]

The medial plantar artery specifically supplies the instep of the foot. The angiosome boundary is the distal medial aspect of the plantar heel, midline of the plantar foot, proximal edge of the plantar forefoot, and an arc 2 to 3 cm above the medial glabrous junction.[1]

There are 2 branches from the medial plantar artery: superficial and deep. The superficial branch projects toward the navicular cuneiform joint and traverses along the superior aspect of the cuneiform and first metatarsal. At the distal first metatarsal, the superficial branch dives plantar medial and eventually joins the deep branch of the medial plantar artery and the first plantar metatarsal artery from the lateral plantar artery. The deep branch of the medial plantar artery courses along the medial intermuscular septum located between the flexor digitorum brevis and abductor hallucis muscle. The artery anastomoses with the first plantar metatarsal and distal lateral plantar artery once it passes deep to the flexor tendons at the level of the first metatarsal neck.[1]

The lateral plantar artery supplies the lateral plantar midfoot and forefoot. Boundaries of the lateral plantar artery angiosome include the distal lateral aspect of plantar heel, central raphe of the plantar midfoot, glabrous junction at the medial plantar forefoot and medial distal dorsal forefoot, glabrous junction of the lateral dorsal and plantar foot, and entire plantar forefoot. The lateral plantar artery forms the deep plantar arch and anastomoses with the dorsalis pedis artery located within the first interspace.[1]

The medial calcaneal artery supplies a segment of the medial and plantar heel. This boundary is found at the glabrous junction of the lateral posterior and plantar heel.[1]

The Anterior Tibial Artery

The anterior tibial artery supplies the anterior compart of the lower extremity. Coursing off the popliteal artery at the inferior aspect of the popliteus muscle, the artery pierces the interosseous membrane and enters the anterior compartment of the lower extremity. The artery can be found descending along the anterior membrane located between the tibialis anterior and extensor digitorum longus.[1,2] The vascular boundary in the lower leg up to the ankle includes the medial aspect of the fibula and anterior aspect of the tibia. At the level of the ankle, the artery branches and gives off the lateral and medial malleolar arteries.[1]

The lateral malleolar artery anastomoses with the perforating peroneal artery, whereas the medial malleolar artery anastomoses with the posteromedial artery from the posterior tibial artery. Distal to the ankle, the artery becomes the deep peroneal artery after exiting deep to the extensor retinaculum. The dorsalis pedis artery supplies the dorsal foot.[1]

The Peroneal Artery

Stemming from the posterior tibial artery peroneal trunk, the peroneal artery can be found in the posterior compartment coursing adjacent to the intermuscular septum along the medial aspect of the fibula.[2] The peroneal artery supplies the posterolateral lower extremity, anterolateral ankle, and lateral rearfoot. The angiosome boundary is the central raphe of the Achilles tendon and anterior edge of the lateral compartment of the lower extremity. The artery supplies the deep posterior muscular compartment, fibula, distal lateral soleus, lateral raphe of the Achilles tendon, and the distal two-thirds of the peroneal muscles.[1]

The peroneal artery bifurcates into the anterior perforating and lateral calcaneal branches. The anterior perforating branch pierces through the intermuscular septum. A branch off the anterior perforating peroneal artery travels superiorly supplying the intermuscular septum and anastomoses with the anterior lateral malleolar artery. The peroneal artery specifically supplies the anterolateral aspect of the proximal ankle. The calcaneal branch supplies the plantar and lateral heel.[1]

PERFORATORS OF THE LOWER LEG

Angiosome boundaries provide a framework to help determine incision placement. Respecting these vascular territories is crucial for flap design and reliability.[1,2]

Each of the 3 main arteries of the lower leg have been found to have consistent perforators within 4 intermuscular septa and 3 distinct perforating clusters.[2,3] Perforators of the lower extremity can be found piercing through the deep fascia of the leg in longitudinal rows adjacent to the intermuscular septa. Previously reported studies have documented an average of 3 to 8 perforators originating from the posterior tibial artery and 3 to 7 originating from the peroneal artery.[3] Depending on the septum of the lower extremity, the number of perforators of the anterior tibial artery is variable.[2,3]

Perforators of the Anterior Tibial Artery

Most of the perforators of the anterior tibial artery are located between the tibia, tibialis anterior, extensor digitorum longus, and peroneus longus (**Fig. 2**). Although there are double the number of perforators present from the anterior tibial artery compared with the peroneal and posterior tibial arteries, the perforator vessel diameters tend to be the smallest. The largest diameter perforators of the anterior tibial artery are found proximally between 3 septa: the tibia and tibialis anterior muscle, extensor digitorum longus and peroneus longus, and the tibialis anterior and extensor digitorum longus.[2,3] Perforators that are located next to the tibia anastomose with posterior tibial perforators present along the tibial surface. As the artery travels distally, the perforator diameters decrease. Schaverien and Saint-Cyr[3] determined that perforators larger than 0.5 cm in diameter were typically found 4 and 9 cm proximal to the ankle joint and located between the tibia and tibialis anterior, or between the tibialis anterior and extensor digitorum longus.

Perforators of the Peroneal Artery

Emerging perforators of the peroneal artery differ depending on location within the distal leg. Proximally, perforators pierce the posterior peroneal septum and can be found coursing through the soleus, or peroneus longus muscle. Distally, perforators are located between the flexor hallucis longus and peroneus brevis (**Fig. 3**). Most peroneal artery perforators are located in the middle third of the fibula. Clusters are located approximately 13 and 18 cm proximal to the ankle joint. The peroneal and posterior tibial perforators anastomose distally at the tendoachilles.[2,3]

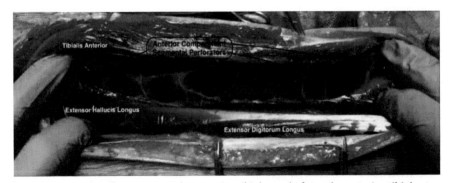

Fig. 2. Segmental perforators over the anterior tibial muscle from the anterior tibial artery. (*From* Ward KL, Romano, A, Rodriguez-Collazo E. Cadaveric Atlas for orthoplastic lower limb and foot reconstruction of soft tissue defects. Clin Surg.2001;3(1); with permission.)

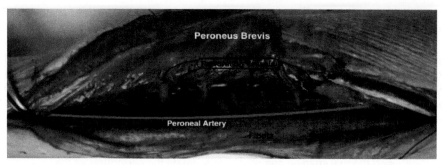

Fig. 3. Peroneal brevis muscle flap perforating vessels branching from the peroneal artery. (*From* Ward KL, Romano, A, Rodriguez-Collazo E. Cadaveric Atlas for orthoplastic lower limb and foot reconstruction of soft tissue defects. Clin Surg.2001;3(1); with permission.)

Perforators of the Posterior Tibial Artery

Superficial and deep perforating arteries originate from the posterior tibial artery supplying the skin and musculature of the lower extremity. Perforators of the posterior tibial artery are the largest in diameter. Most of these perforators are located in the middle third of the leg within the septocutaneous layer and located between the flexor digitorum longus and soleus muscle.[2] Variable perforators of the artery can be found in the peroneal septum. Consistent perforators are present 4 to 9 cm, 13 to 18 cm, and 21 to 26 cm proximal to the ankle joint (**Fig. 4**).[3]

CLINICAL APPLICATION
Preoperative Vascular Evaluation

Preoperative vascular evaluation is strongly advised for planning orthoplastic reconstructive procedures because it dictates the surgical plan and can determine whether vascular anomalies are present.[4–6]

Handheld Doppler
Handheld Doppler has been useful in identifying perforators of the lower extremity. Doppler is able to determine the direction of blood flow but is not able to distinguish

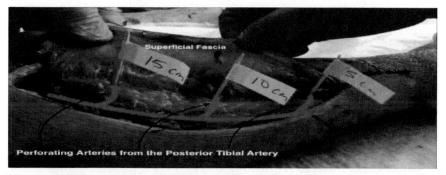

Fig. 4. Medial gastrocnemius and medial soleal flap. Perforators from the posterior tibial artery at 5, 10, and 15 cm piercing through the muscle bellies of the triceps surae into the subcutaneous tissue. Identified with Doppler preoperatively. (*From* Ward KL, Romano, A, Rodriguez-Collazo E. Cadaveric Atlas for orthoplastic lower limb and foot reconstruction of soft tissue defects. Clin Surg.2001;3(1); with permission.)

vessel size or flow volume.[5] A prior understanding of perforator anatomy is necessary and there is variability with this modality because it is operator dependent.[3,5]

Infrared camera

Knowledge regarding venous perforator drainage can be just as important as arterial perforators for flap viability. Fasciocutaneous flaps are reliant on venae comitantes for venous drainage. Infrared cameras are capable of accurately visualizing venous and arterial perforators and can be used preoperative and intraoperative, allowing more freedom in perforator flap design (**Fig. 5**). Venous flow has a higher temperature than arterial flow, making it easy to distinguish perforators from each system.[6] A study by Paul[6] used thermal imaging cameras to investigate the perforators of the lower extremity and found perforator clusters that corresponded with prior reliable perforator locations discussed earlier in this article. To have the best results while using this device it is important to know the working distance, parameters, and thermal range of your specific device.[6]

Computed tomography angiography

Computed tomography angiography (CTA) is a series of high-resolution images of the arterial and venous systems and produces a three-dimensional (3D) reconstruction of soft tissue and bones.[5] Bhattacharya and colleagues[4] evaluated lower extremity perforators with CTA with 3D reconstruction and intraoperative evaluation. They showed that 3D reconstruction with bone incorporation provides exact visualization of perforators as well as their direction and size.[6] With soft tissue and bone incorporation, the vascular continuity can be seen up to the subdermal plexus.[4] CTA provides

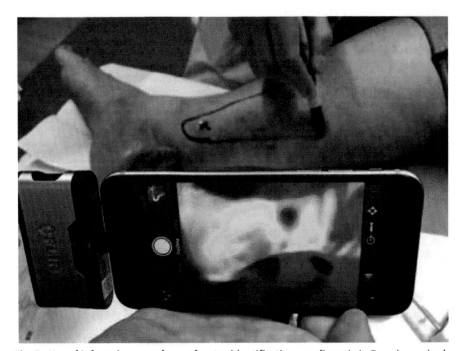

Fig. 5. Use of infrared camera for perforator identification, confirmed via Doppler and subsequent flap design.

valuable insight into perforator anatomy; the diameter, number, and distance from osseous landmarks; and location within the subdermal plexus.[4-6]

CLINICS CARE POINTS

- Each artery within the lower extremity lies within a distinct angiosome boundary.
- The 3 main arteries of the lower leg have consistent perforators present within 4 intermuscular septa and 3 distinct perforating clusters.
- Handheld Doppler, infrared cameras, and CTA are modalities commonly used in preoperative vascular evaluation for planning orthoplastic reconstructive procedures.

DISCLOSURE

The authors declare that they have no relevant or material financial interests that relate to the research described in this article.

REFERENCES

1. Attinger C, Evans K, Bulan E, et al. Angiosomes of the foot and ankle and clinical implications for limb salvage: reconstruction, incisions, and revascularization. Plast Reconstr Surg 2006;117(SUPPLEMENT):261S–93S.
2. Cohen-Shohet R, McLaughlin M, Kerekes D, et al. Evolution of local perforator flaps in lower extremity reconstruction. Plast Aesthet Res 2019;5:28, http://dx.doi.org/10.20517/2347-9264.2019.030.
3. Schaverien M, Saint-Cyr M. Perforators of the lower leg: analysis of perforator locations and clinical application for pedicled perforator flaps. Plast Reconstr Surg 2008;122(1):161–70.
4. Bhattacharya V, Agrawal N, Chaudhary G, et al. CT angiographic evaluation of perforators in the lower limb and their reconstructive implication. Indian J Plast Surg 2012;45(03):494–7.
5. Lee GK, Fox PM, Riboh J, et al. Computed tomography angiography in microsurgery: indications, clinical utility, and pitfalls. Eplasty 2013;13:e42.
6. Paul S. Using a thermal imaging camera to locate perforators on the lower limb. Arch Plast Surg 2017;44(3):243–7.

Medial Plantar Artery Flap for Wound Coverage of the Weight-Bearing Surface of the Heel

Michael D. Liette, DPM[a],
Mohamed A. Ellabban, MD, MBBCh, MSc, MRCS[b],
Pedro Rodriguez, MD[c], Christopher Bibbo, DO, DPM[d],
Suhail Masadeh, DPM[e],*

KEYWORDS

- Ulceration • Neuropathy • Diabetes • Fasciocutaneous flap • Neurocutaneous
- Lower-limb reconstruction

KEY POINTS

- The weight-bearing surface of the foot has a unique anatomy with highly specialized functional units capable of withstanding elevated pressures and unique forces.
- Loss of the specialized anatomy owing to ulceration leads to an increased likelihood of further ulceration and complications.
- Replacing like tissue with like tissue produces a desirable outcome of a stable soft tissue envelope that is more able to withstand pressure and shear forces.
- Tissue from the non–weight-bearing portion of the medial plantar longitudinal arch provides the same specialized anatomy as the heel fat pad.
- The medial plantar artery flap may be designed to provide protective sensation to the weight-bearing portion of the heel.

[a] University of Cincinnati Medical Center, 231 Albert Sabin Way, ML 0513, Cincinnati, OH 45276, USA; [b] Suez Canal University Hospitals and Medical School, Ismailia 41522, Egypt; [c] Plastic and Reconstructive Surgery, OSF Saint Anthony Medical Center, 698 Featherstone Road, Rockford, IL 61107, USA; [d] Foot & Ankle, Reconstructive Plastic & Microsurgery & Limb Salvage, Musculoskeletal Infection & Orthopaedic Trauma, Rubin Institute for Advanced Orthopaedics, International Center for Limb Lengthening, Sinai Hospital of Baltimore, 2401 West Belvedere Avenue, Baltimore, MD 21215-5216, USA; [e] University of Cincinnati Medical Center, Cincinnati Veteran Affairs Medical Center, 231 Albert Sabin Way, ML 0513, Cincinnati, OH 45276, USA
* Corresponding author.
E-mail address: masadesb@uc.edu

Clin Podiatr Med Surg 37 (2020) 751–764
https://doi.org/10.1016/j.cpm.2020.06.002
0891-8422/20/Published by Elsevier Inc.

podiatric.theclinics.com

INTRODUCTION

The plantar skin, much like the palmar skin, has unique properties to resist shear and axial forces. The weight-bearing surface of the heel possesses a unique structure composed of highly specialized fat, compartmentalized by fibrous septae, as seen in **Fig. 1**.[1–3] Tissue loss in this area remains a difficult clinical and surgical problem; because heel wounds have shown significant morbidity and mortality for patients, they occur relatively commonly, and they are often seen with high rates of pursuant osteomyelitis and amputation.[4–7] It is paramount to cover these deficits quickly with a long-term solution to prevent future ulceration and eventual loss of limb. To address this type of tissue loss, the medial plantar artery fasciocutaneous flap serves as a good alternative to other measures.[3,8–13] This specialized flap has the ability to replace "like-with-like" tissue by harvesting the specialized tissue from the more expendable arch of the foot and placing it in the direct weight-bearing plantar heel, which is a high demand area. Furthermore, soft tissue coverage with the medial plantar artery flap is capable of providing protective sensation to the plantar heel.

MEDIAL PLANTAR ARTERY ANATOMY

The posterior tibial artery serves as the source arterial supply of the plantar foot, because it courses retromalleolarly, beneath the flexor retinaculum to enter the plantar foot through the porta pedis. The posterior tibial artery divides into the 2 main divisions, the medial and lateral plantar arteries, along its course beneath the flexor retinaculum, as seen in **Fig. 2**. This branching often occurs before entry into the porta pedis, with the medial plantar artery located superior to the interfascicular ligament and the lateral plantar artery located inferior, within their respective fibrous tunnels, as seen in **Fig. 3**.[14] Several anatomic studies have evaluated the location of the division into the medial and lateral branches and found that this routinely occurs approximately 3 cm distal to the tip of the anterior colliculus of the medial malleolus, at the

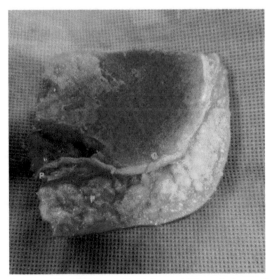

Fig. 1. Sectioned calcaneus (C), with specialized fat pad (F), and plantar fascia (P) consisting of compartmentalized fat pad, separated by thickened fibrous septae. (*Courtesy of* S. Masadeh, DPM, Cincinatti, OH.)

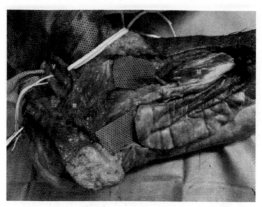

Fig. 2. The structures within the tarsal canal, including the posterior tibial artery (*white vessel loop*), the posterior tibial vein (V), and the posterior tibial nerve (*yellow vessel loop*) as they course beneath the flexor retinaculum (R) to enter the plantar foot deep to the abductor hallucis muscle (M) within the porta pedis. (*Courtesy of* S. Masadeh, DPM, Cincinatti, OH.)

posterior edge of the sustentaculum tali.[8,14,15] The medial plantar artery then travels deep within the intermuscular septum within the medial compartment of the foot, between the flexor digitorum brevis and the abductor hallucis muscles, medial to the flexor hallucis longus tendon, accompanied by the medial plantar nerve.[14] The artery then continues on to divide at the level of the navicular tuberosity, approximately 2.5 to 3.5 cm distal from the medial plantar artery origin, into a deep (medial), superficial (lateral), and a small articular branch, as seen in **Fig. 4**.[16,17] This division has an extremely variable pattern as shown by Macchi and colleagues.[18] In their cadaveric study of 13 specimens, they found a large superficial and small deep branch (type A) with a frequency of 54%, a superficial branch only (type B) with a frequency of 38%, and a large deep branch with a small superficial branch (type C) with a frequency of 8%.

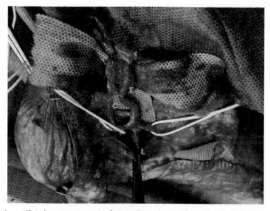

Fig. 3. The posterior tibial artery as it branches into the medial (*white vessel loop*) and lateral (*yellow vessel loop*) plantar arteries before entrance into the porta pedis, separated into fibrous tunnels by the interfascicular ligament (L). Also visualized is the medial calcaneal artery (C) branching off of the posterior tibial artery (T), before entrance into the porta pedis. (*Courtesy of* S. Masadeh, DPM, Cincinatti, OH.)

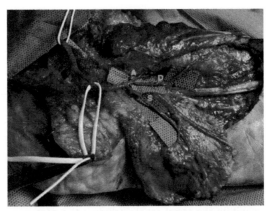

Fig. 4. The arterial anatomy of the medial plantar artery (*white vessel loop*) as it branches from the posterior tibial artery (*yellow vessel loop*). An additional division, occurring at the level of the navicular tuberosity, into the articular branch (A), the deep branch of the medial plantar artery (D), and the superficial branch of the medial plantar artery (S). The superficial branch of the medial plantar artery (S) and the medial plantar nerve (N) is visualized within the elevated fasciocutaneous flap. This highlights an often-tedious area of dissection to ensure incorporation of the dominant pedicle within the flap beneath the navicular tuberosity. (*Courtesy of* S. Masadeh, DPM, Cincinatti, OH.)

After the division into superficial and deep branches beneath the navicular tuberosity, several perforators arise from both of the divisions to provide the cutaneous domain of the flap margins. An average of 3 to 4 septocutaneous perforators arise from the superficial medial plantar artery before its termination in the dense anastomotic network of the first web space, as visualized in **Fig. 5.**[14,17,19] These perforators are highly variable in location along the course of the source artery. A cadaveric study performed by Gao-Men and colleagues[20] found a reproducible perforator at

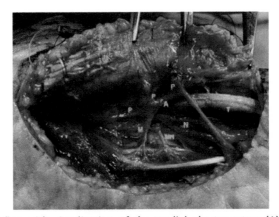

Fig. 5. Elevated flap with visualization of the medial plantar artery (A) and the medial plantar nerve (N) within the flap margins, 3 septocutaneous perforators (P) branching from the medial plantar artery, a muscular branch to the flexor digitorum brevis (M), the motor branch to the flexor digitorum brevis (MN), and the flexor hallucis longus tendon (T) with sheath intact. (*Courtesy of* S. Masadeh, DPM, Cincinatti, OH.)

approximately 2.5 cm from the medial plantar artery origin, termed the middle perforator. The deep branch of the medial plantar artery is further divided into medial and lateral branches and contains a high level of uncertainty regarding its presence and anatomic course. The medial branch travels between the abductor hallucis and the osseous structures of the foot, providing several highly variable perforating branches along its course toward an eventual anastomosis with the first plantar metatarsal artery.[20–22] The lateral branch travels deeper within the foot to its eventual anastomosis with the deep plantar arch and is an unreliable source of perforators for flap design and harvest.

SURGICAL TECHNIQUE

Elevation of the medial plantar artery fasciocutaneous flap requires meticulous dissection and understanding of the anatomy to ensure incorporation of the dominant axial vessel within the flap. Given the high level of variability of the medial plantar artery and its divisions as it traverses the foot, it is important to visualize the artery at the distal most aspect of the flap to ensure inclusion and flap viability at the completion of the procedure.

Before the patient arrives in the operating room, patency of the medial plantar artery must be established via Doppler examination, and if any concerns arise, a preoperative computed tomography angiogram may be performed.[9] The course of the posterior tibial artery and the medial plantar artery should be outlined preoperatively, to further aid in dissection, as seen in **Figs. 6** and **7**.[9] Flap margins are outlined to provide a guide or template, with margins of the flap ideally exceeding the margins of the defect by 1 cm on all sides to prevent excessive tension during flap inset. The medial margin of the flap is not to exceed the level of the navicular tuberosity, and the lateral margin is limited to the most lateral non–weight-bearing portion of the medial longitudinal arch. The proximal margin is the distal portion of the calcaneal tuberosity, and the distal margin is limited to approximately 1 to 2 cm proximal to the metatarsal heads, to avoid the weight-bearing surfaces of the plantar foot, as seen in **Figs. 6** and **7**.[8]

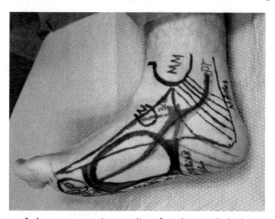

Fig. 6. Medial view of the preoperative outline for the medial plantar artery flap using Doppler examination to identify the course of the artery. Landmarks include the medial malleolus (MM), the navicular tuberosity (N), the Achilles tendon, and the abductor hallucis muscle. The branching point of the medial plantar artery is highlighted in red, approximately 3 cm distal to the medial malleolus beneath the flexor retinaculum, accompanied by the medial plantar nerve and venae comitantes. (*Courtesty of* S. Masadeh, DPM, Cincinatti, OH.)

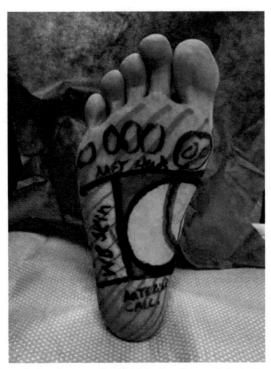

Fig. 7. Plantar view of the preoperative outline for the medial plantar artery flap using Doppler examination to follow the course of the artery as it traverses the plantar foot. The weight-bearing surface, including the metatarsal heads, the lateral column, and the calcaneal tubercle, is identified with orange striping. The margins of the flap are restricted to the non–weight-bearing medial longitudinal arch and are outlined in blue, incorporating the medial plantar artery, nerve, and venae comitantes within the flap. (*Courtesy of* S. Masadeh, DPM, Cincinatti, OH.)

Careful dissection is performed first at the distal margin of the flap, taking care to elevate the plantar fascia from the immediately underlying flexor digitorum brevis muscle and to avoid transection of the long flexor tendons as well as any crossing nerves. By beginning dissection distally, it allows for direct visualization of the dominant pedicle and ensures incorporation with the accompanying venae comitantes and nerve within the flap after elevation. The medial plantar artery and nerve are then isolated deep within the intermuscular septum, located between the abductor hallucis and the flexor digitorum brevis muscles, often lateral to the flexor hallucis longus tendon. The artery is then transected at the distal margin and elevated within the flap while attempting to preserve the medial plantar nerve to retain sensation to the forefoot. The plantar hallucal branch of the medial plantar nerve may be split in an attempt to preserve sensation to the forefoot as well as to restore protective sensation to the heel if so desired.[9,10]

Dissection is then further carried out both medially and laterally along flap margins, elevating the periphery of the flap. Medial dissection is performed overlying the abductor hallucis muscle, taking care to leave the peritendinous structures intact, using the distal tendinous portion as a reference for orientation and further elevation, as seen in **Fig. 8**. Caution must be taken while at the level of the navicular tuberosity,

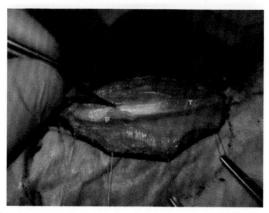

Fig. 8. The medial incision is made using the abductor hallucis tendon (T) as a landmark. Sutures placed through the skin and the fascia are used for atraumatic traction and to prevent avulsion of the deep fascia from the skin. During dissection, it is important to preserve the peritendinous structures (P) overlying the abductor hallucis to maintain a vascularized wound bed for later skin grafting, as seen grasped within the forceps. (*Courtesty of* S. Masadeh, DPM, Cincinatti, OH.)

because of the extensive venous plexus and the variable branching pattern of the superficial and deep branches of the medial plantar artery to avoid isolation of the incorrect arterial supply and loss of incorporation of the pedicle within the flap. Lateral dissection is performed on the lateral-most portion of the medial longitudinal arch, while avoiding the weight-bearing surface of the lateral column. The incision is deepened to the plantar fascia and is elevated off of the underlying flexor digitorum brevis muscle, as seen in **Fig. 9**. During dissection in this area, a higher content of fat is often

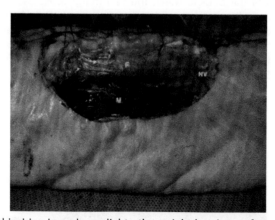

Fig. 9. The lateral incision is made medial to the weight-bearing surface of the lateral column and often has a higher content of fat as one transitions toward the weight-bearing surface. The incision is deepened until the plantar fascia (F) is encountered, taking care to retract any crossing nerves. The plantar fascia is then further elevated off of the underlying flexor digitorum brevis muscle (M), monitoring for the change in consistency of the fat, in which one will encounter the medial plantar neurovascular bundle (NV). (*Courtesty of* S. Masadeh, DPM, Cincinatti, OH.)

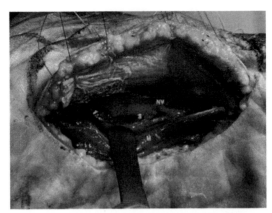

Fig. 10. Further blunt dissection is performed laterally with a pickup to sweep the flexor digitorum brevis muscle (M) down and to identify the septum (S) and the neurovascular bundle (NV) within it. (*Courtesy of* S. Masadeh, DPM, Cincinatti, OH.)

encountered as the transition toward the weight-bearing surface is made. Further dissection is then made bluntly, sweeping the flexor digitorum brevis muscle down to visualize the septum and the medial neurovascular bundle between the medial and central compartments, as seen in **Figs. 10** and **11**. After elevating the distal, medial, and lateral borders, attention is directed proximally to expose the posterior tibial artery beneath the flexor retinaculum. After following the posterior tibial artery to the division of the medial and lateral plantar arteries, the proximal portion of the abductor hallucis tendon is transected, and the medial plantar artery and nerve are exposed within the superior tunnel created by the interfascicular ligament within the porta pedis. Through careful dissection, the artery is followed as it travels distally, allowing for complete exposure of the arterial network of the medial plantar artery and incorporation of the pedicle within the flap margins. Release of the extensive fascial attachments is then performed to allow for an uninhibited arc of rotation and to minimize the potential of kinking during rotation of the flap to cover the heel deficit, as seen in **Figs. 12** and **13**. After release of surrounding fascial attachments, the medial plantar artery flap is freed for rotation into the heel deficit for inset, as seen in **Figs. 14** and **15**.

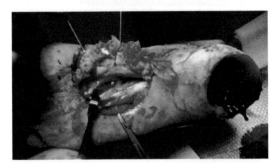

Fig. 11. Lateral dissection with incorporation of the fat pad, the plantar fascia, and the pedicle (P) as well as visualization of the muscular branch to the flexor digitorum brevis. Also seen is the debrided recipient site of the heel, prepared to receive the medial plantar artery flap at the time of inset. (*Courtesy of* S. Masadeh, DPM, Cincinatti, OH.)

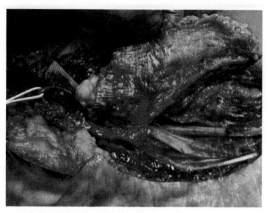

Fig. 12. The septum and the deep fascial attachments (F) to the medial plantar artery flap with incorporation of the superficial branch of the medial plantar artery (A) within the flap margins. (*Courtesy of* S. Masadeh, DPM, Cincinatti, OH.)

LITERATURE REVIEW/RESULTS

There are currently several studies within the literature evaluating the long-term efficacy of the medial plantar artery fasciocutaneous flap for coverage of soft tissue deficits of the heel. The studies evaluated the use of the medial plantar artery–based flap to provide soft tissue coverage for various reasons, including defects created by trauma, malignancy, or neuropathic ulceration. The results of these studies are summarized in **Table 1**.

ANALYSIS/DISCUSSION

Heel decubitus wounds are the second most common ulcer of the lower extremity; covering soft tissue deficits in this area remains challenging because of the specialized anatomy and unique forces at this location.[4] Heel ulcerations have the potential for a high rate of progression to a more proximal amputation because greater than 50% of patients with calcaneal osteomyelitis progress to a below-knee amputation.[7,8]

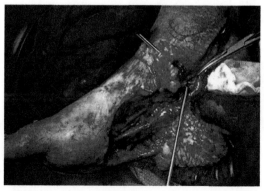

Fig. 13. The deep fascia transection, minimizing kinking potential of the pedicle and allowing for the extensive arc of rotation to transfer the flap for the coverage of the heel soft tissue deficit. (*Courtesy of* S. Masadeh, DPM, Cincinatti, OH.)

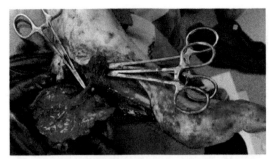

Fig. 14. Fully released and elevated medial plantar artery fasciocutaneous flap with visualized pedicle (P) ready for inset. (*Courtesy of* S. Masadeh, DPM, Cincinatti, OH.)

Therefore, it is critical to cover these deficits quickly to prevent limb loss while maintaining minimal morbidity to the patient.

Because the medial plantar artery is not the dominant artery of the plantar foot, and its angiosome may be perfused by retrograde flow, it is considered to be expendable. The medial plantar artery flap provides coverage for heel ulcers by taking acral tissue from a non–weight-bearing portion of the plantar medial longitudinal arch and rotating it for the coverage of a weight-bearing area.[3,8–13] This flap is able to provide the recipient site with protective sensation and tissues capable of withstanding the higher pressures and shear forces unique to the heel. The presence of numerous fibrous septae connecting deep fascia to skin, high levels of collagen fibers, elastin fibers, and the sealed compartmentalized deposits of fat within the plantar fat pad make the plantar heel anatomy unique.[1–3] These niche characteristics allow for the highly specialized function of the plantar fat pad as a shock absorber.[1,2] The donor site may be readily grafted with either synthetic or autograft at the time of harvest, contingent on the maintenance of a vascularized wound bed at the harvest site, to maintain minimal host

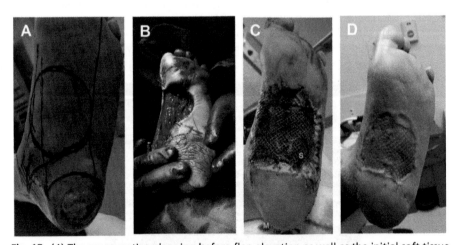

Fig. 15. (*A*) The preoperative planning before flap elevation as well as the initial soft tissue deficit to be covered. (*B*) The initial rotation and inset of the medial plantar artery flap within the heel. (*C*) The split-thickness skin graft (S) placed within the non–weight-bearing portion of the medial longitudinal arch and the healed flap (M). (*D*) The fully healed skin graft and medial plantar artery flap sites. (*Courtesy of* S. Masadeh, DPM, Cincinatti, OH.)

Table 1
Results of medial plantar artery fasciocutaneous flap in the coverage of heel soft tissue deficits

	Number of Patients	Number of Flaps	Average Follow-Up, mo	Ulcer Recurrences (%)	Complications (%)
Okada & Tsukada,[9] 1986	8	8	60	0 (0)	0 (0)
Bibbo,[10] 2012	1	1	24	0 (0)	0 (0)
Mourougayan,[8] 2006	12	12	9–42	0 (0)	0 (0)
Schwarz & Negrini,[11] 2006	48	51	14	7 (14)	5 (10)
Benito-Ruiz et al,[12] 2004	6	6	12–24	0 (0)	1 (17)
Siddiqi et al,[13] 2012	18	18	78	0 (0)	0 (0)
Wann et al,[3] 2011	3	3	12	0 (0)	0 (0)
Total	96	98	9–78	7 (7)	6 (6)

Data from Refs.[3,8–13]

morbidity. The donor site may also be temporized with a dermal regenerative template to improve split-thickness skin graft take and mobility after harvest.

Alternative methods of coverage, such as free flaps and skin grafts, have a higher rate of failure because of lack of highly specialized anatomy and sensation.[23–27] As the heel pad experiences forces up to 80% of body weight during normal weight-bearing and drastic increases in this during heel strike and ambulation, specialized tissues are needed to withstand these forces.[28] Wang and colleagues[29] evaluated the mechanical properties of the heel after reconstruction with various free flaps as compared with intact heel pads. They found a significantly increased energy dissipation ratio, decreased shock absorption, and a loss of elasticity predisposing the free flap to higher levels of heat creation and less elastic recoil. This increased heat production and loss of elasticity has been proposed as a leading factor for repeat ulceration and postoperative complications. Several investigators have reported recurrent ulceration after free tissue transfer to the heel, likely from the combination of sensory deficits and the transplanted tissue not capable of withstanding the forces in this area.[23–27] These studies support the use of a medial plantar artery flap as the primary donor tissue to replace the weight-bearing surface of the heel.

In the senior author's opinion, higher rates of complications may be encountered in patients with diabetes, in patients with severe neuropathy, and in those with a loss of protective sensation. A study performed by Schwarz and Negrini[11] evaluated 51 medial plantar artery flaps in a total of 48 patients with leprosy. They experienced a recurrent ulceration rate of 14% and a complication rate of 5%, notably higher rates in those patients with a total loss of protective sensation because no patients with a functioning medial plantar nerve experienced recurrence.[11] Because many patients are severely neuropathic at the time of tissue loss, they may require protective weight-bearing in an accommodative device or ankle-foot orthotic with a silicone heel for prevention of recurrence later in the postoperative course. In those patients who are sensate, the medial plantar artery flap may be designed to maintain protective sensation. Historically, the technique to maintain protective sensation within the heel has been to transect the medial plantar nerve distally and incorporate this within the flap margins. However, this sacrifices sensation to the plantar medial distal foot and toes, creating further potential postoperative issues through a lack of protective sensation in additional weight-bearing areas. A sensate flap may be created by splitting the plantar hallucal nerve through intraneural, extrafascicular dissection, as described by Bibbo.[10] This technique maintains sensation to the first and second toes while also providing protective sensation to the heel, producing a safer and more effective alternative than transection of the medial plantar nerve distally.

The medial plantar artery fasciocutaneous flap has been proven as a reliable source for soft tissue coverage of heel deficits. It may additionally be used for coverage of various malleolar/ankle or medial foot deficits, but is often reserved for heel ulcerations because of the unique qualities of the flap. It is capable of restoring the functional skin unit of the plantar heel as well as maintaining protective sensation to the weight-bearing surface in those patients without neuropathy, critical to reducing recurrence rates and future complications. Surgical technique and patient selection are also of importance because the variable branching anatomy of the medial plantar artery may prove challenging to ensure the incorporation of the dominant pedicle within the flap margins during harvest. A thorough vascular workup and discussion with the patient about the postoperative course must be performed preoperatively to help ensure improved postoperative outcomes. The overall rate of failures and complications appears to be relatively low, with rates of recurrence reported to be approximately 7% and complication rates of approximately 6% within this review.[3,8–13] These rates are likely lower than can be expected in those patients with diabetes or other complicating factors, such as severe neuropathy, but continue to support the use of this flap in the coverage and management of heel deficits.

CLINICAL CARE POINTS

- Restoring the heel pad is challenging due to the unique functional and structural anatomy of the region.
- Loss of this anatomy leads to an increased likelihood of recurrent ulceration and complications.
- Replacing like tissue with like tissue, capable of withstanding the unique pressure and shear forces in the region, is paramount for successful, durable, and long-lasting outcomes to be achieved.
- Utilizing the tissue from the non-weight bearing portion of the medial longitudinal arch allows for this to occur with only minimal morbidity.
- The medial plantar artery flap may be designed to provide protective sensation to the weight-bearing portion of the heel.

DISCLOSURE

The authors have nothing to disclose.

REFERENCES

1. Jorgensen U, Bojsen-Møller F. Shock absorbency of factors in the shoe/heel interaction—with special focus on role of the heel pad. Foot Ankle 1989;9(11):294–9.

2. Jahss MH, Michelson JD, Desai P, et al. Investigations into the fat pads of the sole of the foot: anatomy and histology. Foot Ankle 1992;13(5):233–42.

3. Wann CD, Gabbay J, Levi B, et al. Quality of innervation in sensate medial plantar flaps for heel reconstruction. Plast Reconstr Surg 2011;127(2):723–30.

4. Barczak CA, Barnett RI, Childs EJ, et al. Fourth national pressure ulcer prevalence survey. Adv Wound Care 1997;10(4):18–26.

5. Boffeli TJ, Collier RC. Near total calcanectomy with rotational flap closure of large decubitus heel ulcerations complicated by calcaneal osteomyelitis. J Foot Ankle Surg 2013;52:107–12.
6. Evans KK, Attinger CE, Al Attar A, et al. The importance of limb preservation in the diabetic population. J Diabetes Complications 2011;25(4):227–31.
7. Faglia E, Clerici G, Caminiti M, et al. Influence of osteomyelitis location in the foot of diabetic patients with transtibial amputation. Foot Ankle Int 2013;34(2):222–7.
8. Mourougayan V. Medial plantar artery (instep flap) flap. Ann Plast Surg 2006; 56(2):160–3.
9. Okada T, Tsukada S. Coverage of heel defects by musculocutaneous and fasciocutaneous flap based on medial plantar neurovascular bundle. Eur J Plast Surg 1986;9:117–21.
10. Bibbo C. Plantar heel reconstruction with a sensate plantar medial artery musculocutaneous pedicled island flap after wide excision of melanoma. J Foot Ankle Surg 2012;51:504–8.
11. Schwarz RJ, Negrini JF. Medial plantar artery island flap for heel reconstruction. Ann Plast Surg 2006;57(6):658–61.
12. Benito-Ruiz J, Yoon T, Guisantes-Pintos E, et al. Reconstruction of soft-tissue defects of the heel with local fasciocutaneous flaps. Ann Plast Surg 2004;52(4): 380–4.
13. Siddiqi MA, Hafeez K, Cheema TA, et al. The medial plantar artery flap: a series of cases over 14 years. J Foot Ankle Surg 2012;51:790–4.
14. Kelikian AS, Sarrafian SK. Sarrafians anatomy of the foot and ankle, 3rd edition. Philadelphia: Lippincott Williams & Wilkins. p. 326–36.
15. Cormack GC, Lamberty BGH. The arterial anatomy of skin flaps. Edinburgh (Scotland): Churchill Livingstone; 1994.
16. Adachi B, Hasebe K. Daigaku Igakubu. Das Arteriensystem der Japaner. Kyoto: Verlag der Kaiserlich-Japanischen Universitat zu Kyoto, in kommission bei. Maruzen Co; 1928.
17. Rodriguez-Vegas M. Medialis pedis flap in reconstruction of palmar skin defects of the digits. clarifying the anatomy of the medial plantar artery. Ann Plast Surg 2007;72(5):542–52.
18. Macchi V, Tiengo C, Porzionato A, et al. Correlation between the course of the medial plantar artery and the morphology of the abductor hallucis muscle. Clin Anat 2005;18:580–8.
19. Orbay H, Kerem M, Unlu RE, et al. Vascular anatomy of plantar muscles. Ann Plast Surg 2007;58(4):420–6.
20. Gao-Men Z, Ahmed Syed S, Tsu-Min T. Anatomic study of a new axial skin flap based on the cutaneous branch of the medial plantar artery. Microsurgery 1995;16:144–8.
21. Bertelli JA, Duarte HE. The plantar marginal septum cutaneous island flap: a new flap in forefoot reconstruction. Plast Reconstr Surg 1997;99:1390–5.
22. Koshima I, Urushibara K, Inagawa K, et al. Free medial plantar perforator flaps for the resurfacing of finger and foot defects. Plast Reconstr Surg 2001;107:1753–8.
23. Mathes SJ, McCraw JB, Vasconez LO. Muscle transposition flaps for coverage of lower extremity defects: anatomic considerations. Surg Clin North Am 1974;54: 1337–54.
24. Gidumal R, Carl A, Evanski P, et al. Functional evaluation of nonsensate free flaps to the sole of the foot. Foot Ankle 1986;7:118–23.
25. Wood MB, Irons GB, Cooney WP. Foot reconstruction by free flap transfer. Foot Ankle 1983;4:2–7.

26. Stevenson TR, Mathes SJ. Management of foot injuries with free-muscle flaps. Plast Reconstr Surg 1986;78:665–71.

27. May JW, Halls MJ, Simon SR. Free microvascular muscle flaps with skin graft reconstruction of extensive defects of the foot: a clinical and gait analysis study. Plast Reconstr Surg 1985;75:627–41.

28. Yucel A, Senyuva C, Aydin Y, et al. Soft tissue reconstruction of sole and heel defects with free tissue transfers. Ann Plast Surg 2000;44:259–69.

29. Wang CL, Shau YW, Hsu TC, et al. Mechanical properties of heel pads reconstructed with flaps. J Bone Joint Surg 1998;81-B:207–11.

First Dorsal Metatarsal Artery Flap for Coverage of Soft Tissue Defects of the Distal Foot

Delayed Technique, Proximal and Distally Based Fasciocutaneous and Adipofascial Variants

Ryan Vazales, DPM[a],*, Suhail Masadeh, DPM[b,1]

KEYWORDS

- First dorsal metatarsal artery flap • Distal soft tissue defects • Distal foot pathology

KEY POINTS

- Coverage options for distal soft tissue defects in the foot remain challenging.
- The first dorsal metatarsal artery flap has several variants, making it a versatile option for challenging distal and proximal foot pathology.
- Delaying the flap may increase flap survival.
- Understanding the variable branching vascular supply for each patient is paramount to flap design and success.

INTRODUCTION

Coverage options for distal soft tissue defects in the foot, in particular digital pathology, is limited. Most of the defects associated with digital or distal foot pathology often are complicated by exposure of tendon or bone, making nonpedicled grafts and random flaps less suitable. Furthermore, split-thickness skin grafts can create unstable scar formation and contracture and even require regrafting.[1] Digital amputation and filet flaps have been described as well but they can alter biomechanical functionality and present morbidity.[2]

[a] Department of Orthopedics, Bon Secours-Mercy Health System, Richmond, VA, USA;
[b] Podiatric Surgery, Veterans Affairs Medical Center, University of Cincinnati, Cincinnati, OH, USA
[1] Present address: 231 Albert Sabin Way, ML 0513, Cincinnati, OH 45276.
* Corresponding author. 7016 Lee Park Road, Suite 105, Mechanicsville, VA 23111.
E-mail address: ryan.vazales@gmail.com

Clin Podiatr Med Surg 37 (2020) 765–773
https://doi.org/10.1016/j.cpm.2020.07.001
0891-8422/20/© 2020 Elsevier Inc. All rights reserved.
podiatric.theclinics.com

The first dorsal metatarsal artery flap (FDMAF) is a less utilized but versatile flap with several variants available for staged reconstruction of soft tissue defects in the foot and digits. It has been utilized to correct tissue defects often caused by traumatic injury, infection, and even tumor resection. These tissue voids create challenges to the limb preservation surgeon because viable, rapid coverage of these areas often is paramount to successful long-term outcomes. The relatively dependable vascular supply, minimal donor site morbidity and functional pliable tissue capable of with-standing Shoe wear make this flap a good option for digital and distal foot defects.[3]

The FDMAF also may be utilized proximally for coverage of soft tissue defects in the midfoot and hindfoot based on the dorsalis pedis arterial (DPA) tree, giving further options for use. The viability of the FDMAF and its variation techniques is predicated on the variable branching vascular supply and perfusion of the superficial network. The existence of a distal communicating arterial branch (DCAB) from the plantar metatarsal artery determines if and what type of flap variants are available for use. Although this flap does not sacrifice a main arterial branch, it may make this flap more suscep-tible to failure with acute transposition along its arc of rotation. For this reason, a delayed method can be utilized to stage the procedure and potentially increase the viability of the flap and provide more reliable successful outcomes.

INDICATIONS

The most common locations for transposition of the FDMAF are digital soft tissue de-fects and distal foot pathology. This flap's multiple variations, however, include adipo-fascial and fasciocutaneous in reverse, propeller-type, and proximal transposition options. The different vascular branching patterns allow for the limits of its indications to be increased.[3] Much of the literature has provided a discussion of noted reasons to undergo the harvest and application of the FDMAF, including traumatic injuries with soft tissue defects; severe infections, including osteomyelitis, which requires both bone and soft tissue resection; failed surgical incisions; tumor resection; and defects to the distal foot that are not amenable for treatment with another flap technique. Furthermore, the flap offers the surgeon an alternative to a free tissue transfer and low donor site morbidity, particularly when utilizing the adipofascial variant.[4]

CONTRAINDICATIONS

Complete contraindications for harvesting the FDMAF are limited but include signifi-cant poor circulation, inability to reach the defect site given its arc of rotation of the flap, too large a tissue deficit, and if another flap with better indication can be utilized. The lack of a DCAB from the plantar metatarsal artery does not preclude utilization of the DFMAF; however, it does determine that a reverse transposition option from prox-imal to distal is not viable.[5]

Relative contraindications continue to evolve as modifications to the technique improve functionality. Relative contraindications for the FDMAF have included pa-tients with 1 or several of the following comorbidities: history of smoking, current smoker, obesity, diabetes, peripheral vascular disease, venous insufficiency/venous outflow disease, and old age.[6]

A vast majority of the literature regarding the FDMAF are case presentations or case series, so the complication rate is variable. Rather than a percentage, literature sug-gests an increased likelihood of failure based on the patient comorbidities and clinical presentation. In higher-risk patient populations, a delayed technique for harvesting of the flap should be considered.

Completing a delayed harvesting technique, the flap is raised over a period of days to weeks. This may ensure the viability of the tissue and may help produce more successful outcomes that also are more reproducible by many different surgeons. The purpose of the delay technique is to improve vascularity and venous outflow to the pedicle prior to acute transposition.

VASCULAR ANATOMY

The vascular supply to the FDMAF is variable, which can be challenging when determining flap design (**Fig. 1**).

The most common origin is the DPA or deep plantar artery, seen in the literature approximately 86% of the time. Otherwise it stems from the plantar circulation or is absent. Its anatomic location, as documented by Lee and Dauber,[7] most often is within a centimeter distal to the medial cuneiform–first metatarsal joint and 5.5 mm plantarward from the dorsal surface of the second metatarsal base. The course of the first dorsal metatarsal artery (FDMA) has variations, as described by Hou and colleagues,[8] relating to is orientation with respect to the first dorsal interosseous muscle belly; although the variant course superficial to the first dorsal interosseous muscle is easier to identify, it is less common then the deeper trek, which travels plantar to the muscle and along the shaft of the first metatarsal. Cutaneous perforators emanate from the FDMA along its course. Aside from scenarios where the FDMA is absent, as it travels distally, it assumes a more superficial position dorsal to the transverse metatarsal ligament before ending in its terminal branches.[8]

The branching pattern of the FDMA as it enters the first digital interspace also is variable. The bifurcation giving off dorsal digital branches to the adjacent toes is not always present. Hou and colleagues[8] identified cases of the digital branches found to only a single digit. Furthermore, preoperative planning utilizing ultrasound color or handheld Doppler identifying the DCAB within the first interspace from the first plantar

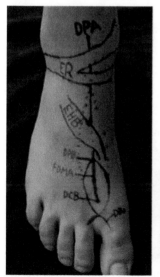
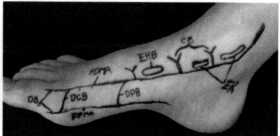

Fig. 1. Vascular supply for the FDMAF, DPA, extensor retinaculum (ER), EHB, deep plantar artery branch (DPB), FDMA, DCAB, FPMA, digital artery branches (DBs), and cutaneous artery branches (CB).

metatarsal artery (FPMA) is paramount to surgical success when utilizing a distally based FDMAF. Although rare, the artery either is absent or too small to provide a viable blood source for a distally based FDMAF in close to 4% of cases.[8] In those cases, transposition distally would not be recommended (**Fig. 2**).

VENOUS CONGESTION

Venous congestion is an important aspect for the correct utilization of any local flap. To deal with this issue, surgeons must take care to establish flap design around a known vascular pedicle. Venous drainage of the reverse flap is supplied by the communicating branches between 2 vena comitantes and collateral branches from each vein or venule, forming a crossover pattern and bypass pattern reverse flow, respectively.[9] Furthermore, venous outflow is critically important for successful management of fluid balance. Venous congestion can inhibit adequate fluid exchange and can lead to ultimate failure.

WHY DELAY TECHNIQUE?

Utilizing the delayed technique and harvesting the pedicle over an extended period of time can increase adequate fluid exchange and decrease likelihood of necrosis that often occurs with a more acute transposition. Delaying the flap improves blood flow to the tissue by increasing vessel size and allowing vessels to undergo reorientation.[10] Furthermore, choke vessels are able to open, increasing perfusion to the flap edges and decrease necrosis.[11] Delay technique is associated with decreased ischemic flap complications in challenging patient populations with significant comorbidities.[12]

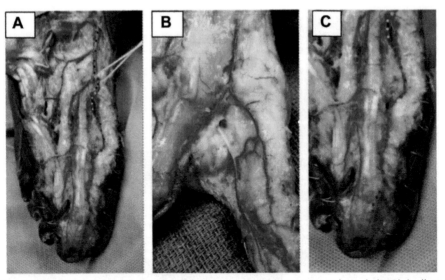

Fig. 2. (*A*) Identification of the DPA (*blue dots*), deep plantar artery branch (DPB) (*yellow dots*), and FDMA (*red dots*). (*B*) FDMA variant with branching digital arteries but no noted DCA from the plantar metatarsal artery. (*C*) DCA (*black dots*), with single digital artery branch.

PATIENT SELECTION AND PREOPERATIVE PLANNING

Strict patient selection criteria always have been an expectation to predict good outcomes. Age, weight, smoking status, vascular status, diabetes mellitus, activity level, and patient goals all have been considered important criteria when choosing a good surgical candidate.

Weight, more specifically obesity, has been a factor in patient selection for localized and distant flap procedures. Obesity is a multifactorial disease consisting of behavioral decisions, environmental factors, and genetic predisposition and has been associated with increased risk of many chronic medical disorders.[13] The increased risk of medical comorbidities associated with obese patient populations often presents a challenge surgically.

The negative effects of active tobacco use, as it relates to increased postoperative complications and poor wound healing, have been well documented within the literature. Furthermore, these findings transcend multiple orthopedic fields and have been supported in arthroplasty, fracture healing, and wound healing research.[14–16]

Diabetes mellitus continues to be a serious growing health concern throughout the world, particularly among surgical candidates, because it has been shown to be associated with poor wound healing and perioperative complications.[17]

Identifying a good surgical candidate followed by an exhaustive preoperative evaluation is key to predicting good surgical outcomes. As discussed previously, most of the defects associated with digital or distal foot pathology often are complicated by exposure of tendon or bone, making nonpedicled grafts and random flaps less suitable. Clinical evaluation is followed by advanced imaging studies, including foot or ankle radiographs and/or magnetic resonance imaging/computed tomography. Treating any and all infections that may be present with a combination of intravenous antibiotics and/or resection of infected bone or tissue should be included as part of the perioperative care. The distally based adipofascial or fasciocutaneous variant of the DFMAF requires that a DCAB from the plantar metatarsal artery be present. The proximally based flap variant does not require a DCAB and still may be a viable option when no DCAB is present. Preoperative confirmation of vasculature is completed utilizing handheld Doppler or color Doppler ultrasound. This includes identification of the DCAB, the FDMA, and DPA.

OPERATIVE TECHNIQUE: A STEPWISE APPROACH
Distally Based Adipofascial and Fasciocutaneous Variants

The patient is placed on the operating table in the supine position. A blanket or bump is placed under the hip, centering the foot and ankle in a perpendicular position to the floor. Once confirmation of vasculature is completed and identification of a DCAB is noted, viability of a distally based FDMAF is confirmed. Flap width generally mirrors that of the defect; however, increasing the length and width of the flap incrementally allows for some atrophy or loss of reach during flap rotation while still covering the defect site without tension.[18] The margins of either the adipofascial or fasciocutaneous flap should be designed in a way that allows the DPA and FDMA to remain centrally within the borders.

A pneumatic tourniquet may be utilized, without limb exsanguination, because this preserves identification of venous structures that should be included. Dissection begins proximally with either a slight lazy S incision or a peninsula incision encompassing the skin paddle and is carried to the level of the DCAB. The proximal vasculature attachments (DPA just inferior to the extensor retinaculum or DBA between the first and second tarsometatarsal joints), based on required arc of rotation, are identified and isolated. The extensor hallucis brevis (EHB) muscle may cross obliquely over the dorsalis pedis and may need to be retracted proximally if necessary. The flap then is carefully elevated just above the extensor tendons, leaving the paratenon intact along the course of the FDMA to the level of the transverse metatarsal ligament distally. Once the flap has been elevated, the tourniquet is deflated and perfusion of the flap is assessed. The dorsalis pedis or deep plantar artery is clamped temporarily (approximately 10–15 mins) and verification that the flap has adequate blood supply from reversed flow FDMA is confirmed.[5]

If adequate perfusion is observed, the proximal vasculature is ligated. Remaining elevation of the flap is completed distally, ensuring that all fibrous attachments surrounding the DCAB have been released to allow unconstrained rotation of the flap at the pivot point. The flap is transposed in a reverse fashion for the adipofascial variant or clockwise/counterclockwise for the fasciocutaneous variant and inset into the defect accordingly. Tunneling of the flap subcutaneously is at the discretion of the surgeon; however, this could increase flap compression and inhibit venous outflow.[4] The literature also has documented dissection of the FDMAF completed from distal to proximal beginning at the pivot point at the level of the DCAB and moving proximally to the DBA or DPA.[18,19] Based on the size of the flap diameter, for adipofascial variants, the donor site is closed primarily when possible under no tension and a split-thickness skin graft from the ipsilateral calf or thigh is harvested and applied to the recipient site of the FDMAF distally.

Proximally Based Adipofascial and Fasciocutaneous Variants

Patient positioning is identical to the distally based variant. Similar to the distally based flap, a handheld or ultrasound Doppler is utilized to identify the FDMA and DPA. The margins of either the adipofascial or fasciocutaneous flap should be designed in a way that allows the DPA and FDMA to remain centrally within the borders. A pneumatic thigh tourniquet may be used.

Dissection begins distally with either a slight lazy S incision for an adipofascial variant or peninsula or island incision encompassing the skin paddle for fasciocutaneous variant. The incision and dissection are carried to the level of the FDMA. The skin or adipofascial paddle is elevated identifying and isolating the subcutaneous fascial pedicle followed by raising the flap and pedicle with the fascia included to the level of the DPA pivot point (**Fig. 3**). Again, the harvested flap should be approximately 1.5-cm larger in diameter then the total defect to account for retraction of the tissues over time. Arterioles can be ligated and cauterized carefully. A fasciocutaneous or adipofascial harvest can be completed and carried the entire length of the pedicle or alternatively the flap may include a fasciocutaneous distal paddle and an entirely adipofascial pedicle proximally to the level of the pivot point. Once the flap is elevated, the tourniquet is deflated and flap perfusion is confirmed, followed by ligation of the distal vasculature prior to insetting the flap into the defect. When the soft tissue defect is noted within the proximal foot or distal ankle area, application of an external fixator device may be utilized to augment flap stabilization.

The donor site often is closed primarily when able under no tension and a split-thickness skin graft or skin substitute graft is placed over the flap proximally.

Delayed technique in proximally or distally based flap design raises the paddle and pedicle in sections and allows a period of days to weeks with the flap reapproximated in the donor site for better adaptation of tissues prior to transposition. The time for delay remains variable within the literature; however, 4 days to 15 days of delay leaving the flap approximated within its donor site prior to transposition is well supported. This time frame can be modified based on the pathophysiology and patient population,

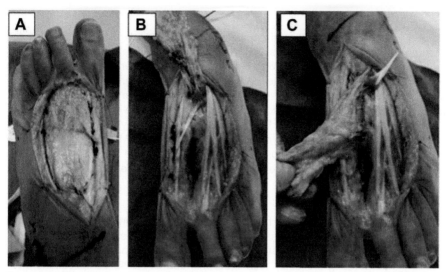

Fig. 3. (*A*) Proximally based adipofascial variant of the FDMAF. Initial adipofascial harvest of the FDMAF. (*B*) Adipofascial variant of the FDMAF with EHB crossing obliquely at the level of the dorsa pedis artery (DPA). (*C*) Adipofascial harvest with resection of the EHB muscle to decrease tension/adhesions and increase arc of rotation of the flap.

delaying for a longer time period in more challenging pathology and significant comorbidity history.[12]

POSTOPERATIVE CARE
Distally Based First Dorsal Metatarsal Artery Flap

When only soft tissue procedures are completed with no bony fusions or osteotomies that augment the procedure, the postoperative course entails immobilization in a soft dressing with protective boot or offloading device for a period of time. Alternatively, a posterior splint or cast may be utilized. This flap rarely requires any type of external fixator because immobilization is maintained with dressings, discussed previously. Time to suture removal is based on surgeon preference but generally is guided by healing of the split-thickness skin graft at either the donor or recipient site when utilized. Transition to a removable walking boot for a short period of time often is part of the postoperative course. These patients may require custom accommodative inserts and shoe gear to maintain an even distribution of weight across the foot and decreased pressure over the flap site.

Proximally Based First Dorsal Metatarsal Artery Flap

Proximal transposition of this flap into the posterior foot and into the distal ankle requires a slightly different postoperative course. Proximally based flaps may be augmented by immobilization with external fixator device, which is left in place until the split-thickness skin graft has healed. Generally, stitches are removed at week 3 followed by scheduling of removal of the external fixator device.

Again, custom shoe gear with inserts may be required, based on patient population. These guidelines for all variants of this flap are general and all dependent on incisional healing.

COMPLICATIONS

Surgeons may encounter several complications when utilizing local tissue transfer, including this procedure. Venous congestion, flap compression, and flap necrosis as well as donor site complications in flap diameters greater than 2.5 cm all have been well documented within the literature. Venous hypertension, associated with subcutaneous veins in distally based flaps that usually engorge and finally thrombose, hindering venous drainage, should be ligated to minimize flap congestion.[20]

The benefits of the adipofascial FDMAF include the ability to yield a larger-sized flap, primary closure of the donor sites on flap diameters less than 2.5 cm, and its versatility in being able to be transferred to a distal or proximal pedicle. A split-thickness skin graft, however, often is needed to cover over the flap at the recipient site.[4]

SUMMARY

A well-planned surgical decision, based on patient selection and extensive preoperative work-up, including vascular assessment, plays a large role in successful postoperative outcomes. Combined with utilizing the best variation of the FDMAF and possibly incorporating the delay technique, this can decrease complications often encountered with the procedure.

CLINICAL CARE POINTS

- The dorsal first metatarsal artery flap can provide stable coverage for forefoot defects allowing the use of regular shoe gear.
- Direct Donor site closure maybe difficult and may require a skin graft for closure.
- Preservation of the extensor tendons sheath can reduce donor site morbidity.
- Inadequate release of fascial constraints surrounding the pedicle can contribute to venous congestion and subsequent failure of the flap.

REFERENCES

1. Yeo CJ, Sebastin SJ, Ho SY, et al. The dorsal metatarsal artery perforator flap. Ann Plast Surg 2014;73:441–4.
2. Emmett AJ. The filleted toe flap. Br J Plast Surg 1976;29:19–21.
3. Serletti JM, Moran SL. Soft tissue coverage options for dorsal foot wounds. Foot Ankle Clin 2001;6:839–51.
4. Senyuva C, Yucel A, Fassio E, et al. Reverse first dorsal metatarsal artery adipofascial flap. Ann Plast Surg 1996;36:158–61.
5. Hayashi A, Maruyama Y. Reverse first dorsal metatarsal artery flap for reconstruction of the distal foot. Ann Plast Surg 1993;31(2):117–22.
6. Whiteford L. Nicotine, CO and HCN: the detrimental effects of smoking on wound healing. Br J Community Nurs 2003;8:S22–6.
7. Lee JH, Dauber W. Anatomic study of the dorsalis pedis-first dorsal metatarsal artery. Ann Plast Surg 1997;38:50–5.
8. Hou Z, Zou J, Wang Z, et al. Anatomical classification of the first dorsal metatarsal artery and its clinical application. Plast Reconstr Surg 2013;132:1028e–39e.
9. Lin SD, Lai CS, Chiu CC. Venous drainage in the reverse forearm flap. Plast Reconstr Surg 1984;74:508–12.
10. Fisher J, Gingrass MK. Basic principles of skin flaps. In: Georgiade GS, Riefkohl R, Levin LS, editors. Plastic, maxillofacial and reconstructive surgery. Baltimore (MD): Williams and Wilkins; 1997. p. 22–4.

11. Dhar SC, Taylar GI. The delay phenomenon: the story unfolds. Plast Reconstr Surg 1999;104:2079–91.
12. Foran MP, Schreiber J, Christy MR, et al. The modified reverse sural artery flap lower extremity reconstruction. J Trauma 2008;64:139–43.
13. Tjepkema M. Adult obesity. Health Rep 2006;17:9–25.
14. Kapadia BH, Issa K, Pivec R, et al. Tobacco use may be associated with increased revision and complication rates following total hip arthroplasty. J Arthroplast 2014;29(4):777–80.
15. Kapadia BH, Johnson AJ, Naziri Q, et al. Increased revision rates after total knee arthroplasty in patients who smoke. J Arthroplast 2012;27(9):1690–5.
16. Mosely LH, Finseth F. Cigarette smoking: impairment of digital blood flow and wound healing in the hand. Hand 1977;9(2):97–101.
17. Tsang ST, Gaston P. Adverse peri-operative outcomes following elective total hip replacement in diabetes mellitus: a systematic review and meta-analysis of cohort studies. Bone Joint J 2013;95B(11):1474–9.
18. Hallock GG. The first dorsal metatarsal artery perforator propeller flap. Ann Plast Surg 2016;76:6.
19. Cheng MH, Ulusal BG, Wei FC. Reverse first dorsal metatarsal artery flap for reconstruction of traumatic defects of dorsal great toe. J Trauma 2006;60(5): 1138–41.
20. Chang SM. Role of large superficial veins in distally based flaps of the extremities. Plast Reconstr Surg 1999;103:494.

Utility of the Digital Fillet Flap

Suhail Masadeh, DPM[a,b,*], Pedro Rodriguez, MD[c], Alec J. Dierksheide, DPM[b], Peter A. Crisologo, DPM[b]

KEYWORDS

• Digital fillet • Filleted flap • Toe fillet • Ulcer • Soft tissue deficit

KEY POINTS

- Coverage options should be durable and reconstruct tissues in a "like with like" fashion to accommodate the high plantar pressures and sheer forces.
- The digital fillet flap provides a valuable option for forefoot soft tissue deficit coverage.
- A careful understanding of the anatomy and patient selection is paramount to achieve optimal outcomes.

INTRODUCTION

Soft tissue reconstruction of plantar forefoot soft tissue deficits is particularly challenging due to the specialized nature of the soft tissue envelope of the foot. These soft tissue deficits predispose patients to infection and places them at a risk for major amputation. For example, more than half of patients with diabetes and a foot wound become infected during treatment, with 20% developing osteomyelitis.[1] The challenge for coverage of a soft tissue deficit in part is secondary to the thin subcutaneous tissue dorsally with superficial tendons, the specialized plantar fat pad with limited mobility, the prominent osseous structures, and the tenuous blood supply of the forefoot. Furthermore, the plantar weight-bearing skin is unique in its ability to dissipate shear and ground reactive forces. Therefore, ideal coverage would follow the concept of replacing "like with like" to ensure durability and sustainably that can withstand the stress of ambulation. With these concepts in mind, one option for coverage is the digital fillet flap.

The digital fillet flap is an axial pattern flap, meaning it has a named source artery, the digital artery. The flap design is variable, pending defect location and the length

[a] Department of Surgery, U.S. Department of Veterans Affairs, Cincinnati VA Medical Center, 3200 Vine Street, Cincinnati, OH 45219, USA; [b] Department of Surgery, Division of Podiatric Surgery, University of Cincinnati Medical Center, 231 Albert Sabin Way, ML 0513, Cincinnati, OH 45276, USA; [c] Plastic and Reconstructive Surgery, OSF Saint Anthony Medical Center, 698 Featherstone Road, Rockford, IL 61107, USA
* Corresponding author. Department of Surgery, Division of Podiatric Surgery, University of Cincinnati Medical Center, 231 Albert Sabin Way, ML 0513, Cincinnati, OH 45276.
E-mail address: Suhail.Masadeh@va.gov

Clin Podiatr Med Surg 37 (2020) 775–787
https://doi.org/10.1016/j.cpm.2020.07.009
0891-8422/20/Published by Elsevier Inc.

podiatric.theclinics.com

of reach needed. The flap can be elevated as a peninsular flap, based on the dorsal or plantar system for local transposition (case 1). An alternative is a neurovascular island flap, as described by Moberg[2] and Littler to achieve greater reach. The flap is incised circumferentially, raised on its pedicle, and inset in a nearby deficit (case 2). Both of these techniques require skin grafting of the donor site. Multiple flaps can also be designed as part of the spare part surgery technique, where soft tissue outlined for amputation is utilized for preservation of length in amputation surgery (case 3). Finally, the digits can be utilized as free flaps, most commonly used for replantation surgery in the hand.

LITERATURE REVIEW

With only a singular systematic review, published 5 years ago, there is a limited amount of information in the literature that currently exists about the outcomes of digital fillet flaps for soft tissue coverage in limb salvage scenarios.[3] The aim of this article is to describe the digital fillet flap and its utility and give updated data on the use of digital fillet flap for soft tissue defects of the foot.

ARTERIAL ANATOMY

The foot is subject to significant mechanical stress and thus is highly prone to injury that can compromise flow. In true form and function fashion, the foot has multiple arterio-arterial connections. The dual blood supply serves as a protective mechanism from ischemia by increasing avenues of collateral blood flow and soft tissue perfusion. Knowledge of the vascular supply of the foot and its variants is crucial for the surgical management of soft tissue deficits and more specifically flap utilization. Within the duality of blood supply, often there is a dominant system of perfusion that is more suitable for tissue harvest.

In the forefoot, the source arteries consist of the dorsalis pedis (DP), medial plantar artery (MPA), and lateral plantar artery (LPA). These systems are intricately connected in the form of arterio-arterial anastomosis.

Each vessel is discussed in more detail (**Fig. 1**).

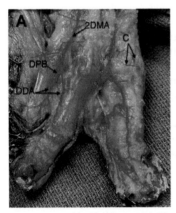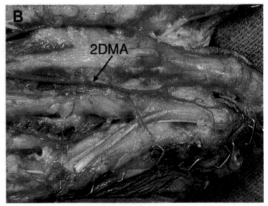

Fig. 1. Anatomy of the digital fillet flap. (*A*) 2DMA, second DMA; C, cutaneous branches; DDA, dorsal digital arteries (to the lateral and medial second and third toes, as depicted); DPB, distal perforating branch, connects dorsal arterial system with the plantar system. (*B*) 2DMA, second DMA; note the cutaneous branches. (*Courtesy of* S. Masadeh, DPM, Cincinnati, OH.)

The DP is the continuation of the anterior tibial artery. It divides into several branches, including the lateral and medial tarsal arteries, arcuate artery, and first dorsal metatarsal artery (FDMA), and communicates with the deep plantar arch via a perforating branch in the first interspace. The DP also gives off multiple direct cutaneous branches to the dorsal foot.

The lateral tarsal artery courses laterally on the dorsal foot deep to the extensor hallucis brevis and extensor digitorum brevis muscles, supplying both muscles.

The FDMA is the continuation of the DP into the first interspace. The FDMA has 3 branches, a medial branch under the extensor hallucis tendon to supply the medial side of the great toe, and, at the level of the metatarsophalangeal joint, its terminal end divides into 2 branches to supply the lateral great toe and medial second toe. The medial branch to the hallux has a larger caliber than its lateral counterpart to the second digit. Distally the FDMA anastomoses with the first plantar metatarsal artery.[4] The FDMA has been studied and used extensively in the hand as a free flap.

The deep plantar arch is formed by the DP and LPA and extends from the first interspace in a convex fashion superficial to the bases of the lesser metatarsals and plantar interosseous muscles and deep to the adductor hallucis muscle. The dep arch divides into 4 plantar metatarsal arteries, which connect to the dorsal metatarsal arteries (DMAs) via perforating branches in the forefoot interspaces proximally and distally.

The plantar metatarsal arteries divide further at the web spaces to supply the sides of the lesser digits via the plantar digital arteries. The first plantar metatarsal artery also gives a branch to supply the medial plantar aspect of the great toe.

The arcuate artery, when present, courses laterally and distally in a convex fashion by the medial cuneiform over the metatarsal bases and it connects with the lateral tarsal artery proximally and with the plantar metatarsal arteries via distal and proximal perforating branches.[5,6] It gives rise to the second, third, and fourth DMAs, which further divide at the web spaces to give off the dorsal digital arteries to supply the sides of the central lesser digits. When the arcuate artery is absent, the second, third, and fourth DMAs arise from the lateral tarsal artery. The fifth digit receives a lateral dorsal artery branch supplied by a branch of the fourth DMA.

The MPA and LPA are the terminal branches of the posterior tibial artery. Both arteries travel into the plantar foot via the porta pedis deep to the abductor hallucis muscle. The lateral plantar is the larger of the 2 branches and travels toward the base of the fifth metatarsal. The MPA travels distally in the foot between the abductor hallucis and flexor digitorum brevis in the medial compartment of the foot.

The MPA is discussed in detail in another article in this issue. For the purpose of this section, The MPA divides into a superficial and deep branch; at the base of the first metatarsal, the deep branch travels toward the medial hallux where it joins the branch of the first plantar metatarsal artery. The superficial branch of the MPA curves in a convex and superficial pattern to form the superficial plantar arch and divides into 3 superficial branches that anastomose with the deep plantar metatarsal arteries to supply the plantar digital arteries.

The LPA passes between the flexor digitorum and abductor digiti minimi toward the base of the fifth metatarsal as it curves medially to join the DP in forming the deep plantar arch, discussed previously. The LPA gives off a direct plantar digital branch to the fifth digit. In certain instances, there is an anastomosis with the MPA and when this is present it forms a superficial plantar arch.

SURGICAL TECHNIQUE

Flap design is dependent on the location and size of the defect and whether a digit is expendable. A handheld Doppler is utilized to identify and mark the course of the digital arteries. The central digits can be approached from dorsal central or plantar central incisions; the hallux and fifth digits can be approached from medial incision or lateral incision, respectively; the dissection is performed under loop magnification. The plane of dissection should be carried in the avascular plane following the extensor tendons. The nail unit is excised, and full-thickness flaps are elevated with care taken to preserve the neurovascular bundle. An arthrotomy is performed at the level of the metatarsal phalangeal joint and the phalanges with their associated extensor and flexor tendons are filleted from the flap without damage to the neurovascular bundle. Intraoperative Doppler is utilized to assess signal of the digital arteries along with the clinical examination of flap edge bleeding. If there are any perfusion problems detected, the authors recommend delay of flap inset. If a strong signal and adequate flap edge bleeding is present, the flap can be inset without tension. Post–flap inset, additional assessment of perfusion is performed, utilizing the handheld Doppler along with capillary fill time to ensure adequate perfusion is present. If the signal is lost or the flap is white, sutures are removed in a systematic fashion until adequate perfusion is noted. If concern of perfusion is still present, the authors recommend placing the flap at the site of harvest and delaying the flap inset. The digital arteries are prone to spasm and, therefore, the authors recommend utilization of antispasmodic medications, such as papaverine or lidocaine, along with warm saline irrigation. This may take up to 15 minutes to resolve prior to making the decision for flap delay.

Table 1
Follow-up and complications reported for pedal digital fillet flaps

Author, Year	Patients (N)	Follow-up (Months)	Complications
Snyder and Edgerton,[7] 1965	2	3	None
Kaplan,[8] 1965	1	NR	Wound dehiscence
Emmett,[9] 1976	1	48	None
Morain,[10] 1984	7	4–42	1 BKA
Lin et al,[11] 2000	9	7–48	1 flap required revision, 1 NSTI requiring BKA 2 y postoperative, 1 ray resection 7 months postoperative
Küntscher et al,[12] 2001	11	NR	18% types of complications
Kalbermatten et al,[13] 2004	1	3	NR
Yarmel et al,[14] 2008	1	5	NR
Aerden et al,[15] 2012	4	12	1 wound dehiscence requiring surgical revision, 3 new ulcers (1 minor amputation, 2 corrective osteotomies)
Eliezer et al,[16] 2017	4	0–5	NR

Abbreviations: BKA, below-knee amputation; NR, not reported; NSTI, necrotizing soft tissue injury.
Data from Refs.[7–16]

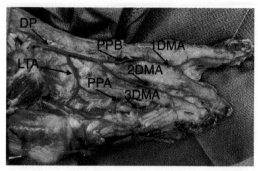

Fig. 2. The arcuate artery is present only 16.7% of the time, whereas the second, third, and fourth DMAs arise from the lateral tarsal artery 47% of the time. 1DMA, FDMA; 2DMA, second DMA; 3DMA, DMA; LTA, lateral tarsal artery; PPA, proximal perforating artery to plantar system—note the absence of the arcuate artery; PPB, proximal perforating branch to deep plantar arch. (*Courtesy of* S. Masadeh, DPM, Cincinnati, OH.)

LITERATURE REVIEW METHODS

This is a review of the current literature and did not require formal ethical approval. No patient information was encountered or handled. A search was performed in PubMed (www.pubmed.gov) and Google Scholar (www.google.com/scholar) up to and including articles published through November 20,2019, using the search terms, digital, flap, fillet flap, filleted flap, or ulcer for both Google Scholar and Pubmed. Articles were required to be published in the English language. A search also was performed of the references of the included texts. Studies then were identified and reviewed by 2 authors (SBM and PAC) for appropriateness; 51 texts were reviewed in full by 2 authors (SBM and PAC) for appropriateness and ultimately.

No restrictions were placed on the cause of the soft tissue deficit, unforeseen complications, or duration of follow-up. The search was performed by AJD and PAC. PAC examined and verified the subject matter of the search in reference to the inclusion criteria, discussed previously, or exclusion criteria of the studies. Additional studies were identified and acquired by examining the relevant studies cited in the reference lists of published research.

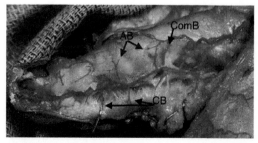

Fig. 3. Hallux arterial system. AB, articular branch to the proximal interphalangeal joint; CB, cutaneous branches; ComB, communicating branch between dorsal and plantar digital arteries. (*Courtesy of* S. Masadeh, DPM, Cincinnati, OH.)

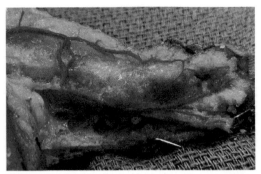

Fig. 4. Note the distal tuft arcade. (*Courtesy of* S. Masadeh, DPM, Cincinnati, OH.)

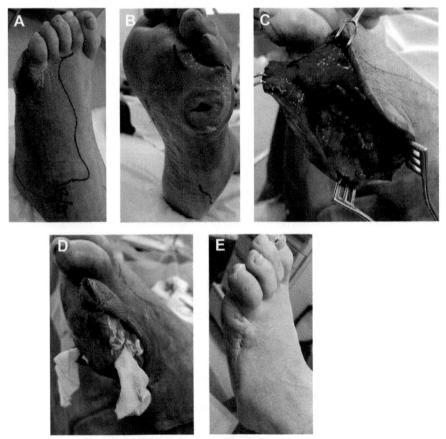

Fig. 5. Case 1, sub–fifth metatarsal ulceration and osteomyelitis. (*A, B*) Diabetic patient with infected plantar ulceration with cellulitis. (*C*) Infection is controlled by excising the infected bone while maintaining soft tissues after fillet of the phalanges via a lateral approach. (*D*) The flap is delayed until the infection is cleared. This process typically is 14 days and is in conjunction with the use of pathogen directed parenteral antibiotic therapy. (*E*) Inset, with complete incorporation of the flap at 3 months. (*Courtesy of* S. Masadeh, DPM, Cincinnati, OH.)

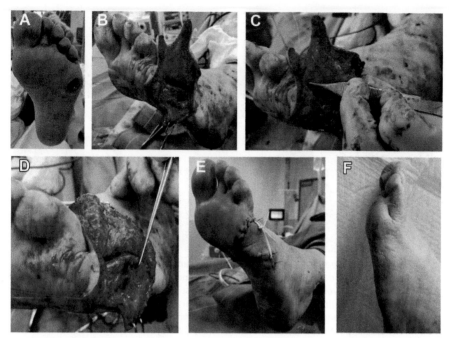

Fig. 6. Case 2, sub–fifth metatarsal ulceration and osteomyelitis. (*A*) Diabetic with plantar sub–fifth metatarsal ulceration with associated osteomyelitis of the fifth metatarsal head. (*B*) Elevation of fifth digit fillet flap and resection of fifth ray; note atraumatic technique for flap elevation. (*C*) Note instrument pointing to the plantar medial digital artery. (*D*) Flexor digiti minimi elevated and transposed to cover the resected margin of the fifth metatarsal. (*E*) Flap inset with vessel loop as a drain to prevent hematoma formation beneath the flap. (*F*) Complete healing and incorporation at 4 weeks and the patient returned to shoes at 3 months. (*Courtesy of* S. Masadeh, DPM, Cincinnati, OH.)

RESULTS

For the review performed in November 2019, by authors AJD and PAC, there were a total number of 10 references were included from the 51 fully reviewed articles.[7–16] Most of the studies that were included were of level III and level IV evidence. Since the last systematic review on this topic published by Schade[3] in 2014, only 2 additional studies met the inclusion criteria for a total of 10 studies.

A total of 40 patients with a mean age of 50.7 years (8–84 years) were included in the search of the literature. Follow-up was reported for only 22 patients and the average was 15.9 months. An array of complications existed but were reported intermittently and aggregate reporting was unable to be done reliably (**Table 1**).

DISCUSSION

The digital fillet flap has been shown to be a versatile procedure in all subtypes, as described by Küntscher and colleagues[12] based on their combined data of 104 fillet flaps (**Figs. 2–10**). This classification was presented to organize the type of fillet flap by the relative extent and technique of the filleted flap (**Table 2**).

In the lower extremity, the digital fillet flap was first described as a neurovascular island free flap, first by Kaplan[8] and Snyder and Edgerton[7] in 1965. Emmett[9] later

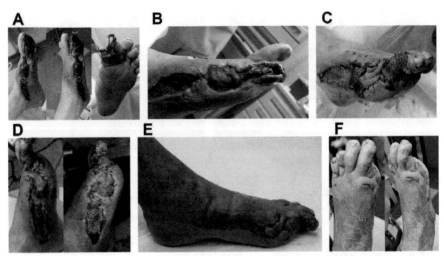

Fig. 7. Case 3, diabetic patient with failed bone block arthrodesis and osteomyelitis. (*A*) Diabetic patient with failed bone block arthrodesis secondary to severe PAD with necrosis of the hallux and osteomyelitis of the phalanges. (*B*) Post-débridement of the wound plantar lateral aspect of the hallux remained viable. (*C*) Dorsal digital artery peninsular fasciocutaneous flap, donor site and remaining deficit covered with split-thickness skin graft. (*D*) One week and 2 weeks postinset. (*E*) Six weeks postinset, delayed healing of donor site; care must be taken to preserve synovial sheath over the extensor tendon; otherwise, the donor site will not accept a skin graft. (*F*) Three months postoperative, complete healing of donor site with incorporation of flap and skin graft. (*Courtesy of* S. Masadeh, DPM, Cincinnati, OH.)

described a type A1 (see **Table 2**) digital fillet flap in a case report, where he sacrificed the third toe for coverage of a plantar forefoot weight-bearing area where the patient had previously failed local wound care and a split-thickness skin graft. He found this to be a successful procedure with a 4-year follow-up of the patient without breakdown or complication.[9]

Morain[10] expanded on the work of Kaplan,[8] Snyder and Edgerton,[7] and Emmett[9-] with a 7-patient case series of both type A1 and type A2 digital fillet flaps. Morain[10] was the first to describe complications beyond wound dehiscence associated with type A fillet flaps with 1 patient who underwent a below-knee amputation secondary to sepsis, 1 reulcerated, and another had flap failure. Although Morain[10] was the first to publish a case series, it is difficult to draw definitive conclusions, given only 7 patients were included and there was a combination of different digital fillet subtypes.

Lin and colleagues[11] published the next case series of 9 filleted toe flaps, which included a combination of etiologies, including not only patients with diabetes (n = 4) but also posttraumatic patients (n = 2) and patients with ischemic wounds (n = 3). Lin and colleagues[11] reported similar rates of complications as Morain[10] did, including 1 flap failure secondary to infection requiring revisional ray amputation and skin grafting and recurrent infection at the site of filleted digit flap requiring the ray to be amputated for resolution. Lin also reported 1 below-knee amputation but this was unrelated to the index digital fillet procedure because this occurred 2 years after the patient healed and was secondary to an unrelated necrotizing soft tissue infection.[11]

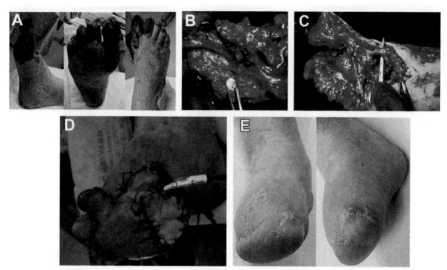

Fig. 8. Case 4, patient with diabetes and tissue loss secondary to PAD. (*A*) Diabetic with gangrene status post-revascularization; note preserved web space and lateral skin island to the great toe and plantar skin of the second digit. (*B*) Fillet of the great toe and second toe; note plantar lateral digital artery. (*C*) Note the dorsal first metatarsal artery. (*D*) Lateral hallux was inset plantarly and the second digit was inset dorsally over the hallux. A small section of the flap was de-epithelialized inferior to the second digit fasciocutaneous flap. The remaining digits were also filleted, left intact, and later used as full-thickness skin graft to cover a decubitus heel ulcer and lateral ankle ulcer. (*E*) Three months postoperative noted complete healing of the flaps and TMA. PAD, peripheral arterial disease; TMA, transmetatarsal amputation. (*Courtesy of* S. Masadeh, DPM, Cincinnati, OH.)

Kalbermatten and colleagues[13] published a variation of a type A1 digital fillet flap, where they described a double toe fillet flap in a patient with diabetes and a partial forefoot amputation. This involved sacrificing a nonfunctional fourth toe and the tissue was divided. The distal portion of the flap was de-epithelialized (including the extensor tendon) and used as a vascularized extensor tendon complex and used for a soft tissue filler and the proximal portion of the flap of the fourth toe then was used for skin coverage.[13] The digital fillet also has been described in the pediatric population as a case study from recurrent hemangioendothelioma resection in an 8-year-old patient by Yarmel and colleagues,[14] using the second toe for coverage of a first interspace deficit.

Since the systematic review by Schade,[3] there have been 2 more case series published.[15,16] Aerden and colleagues,[15] reported 4 cases, where the hallux was used to assist with closure of transmetatarsal amputations in patients with diabetic foot infections, with a mean healing time of 44 days and a 12-month follow-up. In the 4 cases where the hallux was filleted, Aerden and colleagues[15] reported only 1 immediate postoperative complication in which there was a persistent wound dehiscence, where a drain was placed and ultimately required surgical revision to allow for closure. After the initial perioperative period, 3 (75%) of the patients developed transfer ulcerations, requiring 1 minor amputation and 2 corrective osteotomies.[15] Eliezer and colleagues[16] reported a case series to similar that of Aerden and colleagues[15] of 4 patients with diabetes, where the hallux and remaining medial foot tissue were used to provide soft

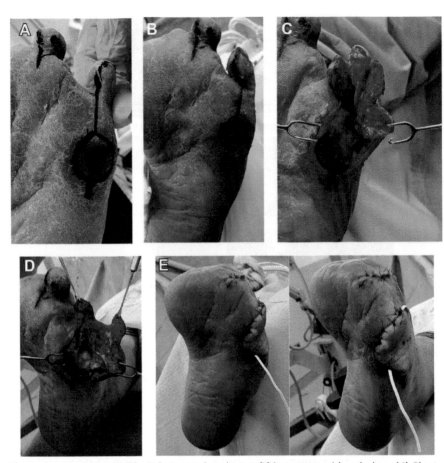

Fig. 9. Case 5, patient with diabetes and a plantar fifth metatarsal head ulcer. (*A*) Plantar ulcer with osteomyelitis of the fifth metatarsal head. (*B*) Full-thickness excision of the ulcer. (*C*) Fifth digit fillet flap from plantar approach. (*D*) The phalanges disarticulated at the fifth MTPJ and filleted from the soft tissue. (*E*) Flap inset. MTPJ, metatarsal phalangeal joint. (*Courtesy of* S. Masadeh, DPM, Cincinnati, OH.)

tissue coverage of transmetatarsal amputations. Unlike Aerden and colleagues,[15] Eliezer and colleagues[16] had shorter follow-up (0–5 months) and did not report complications.

When dealing with patients with foot ulcerations, they often are complicated by diabetes. The patient with diabetes and a foot ulceration is at a greater than 50% risk of infection.[1] Of these patients who become infected, approximately half of these require a partial foot amputation and 10% required a proximal amputation.[17] Given these risks, it is judicious to consider options for early coverage and wound healing in these high-risk patients. The potential risks and benefits should be discussed with the patient when making a decision to fillet a digit from a grossly stable digit for coverage of a deficit or salvage of another digit, such as with a free transfer to the hand.[18–20]

The utility of the digital fillet flap in the foot has become an increasingly popular option for management of deficits not amenable to primary closure. Since they were first described by Snyder and Edgerton[7] in 1965 as a neurovascular island flap for

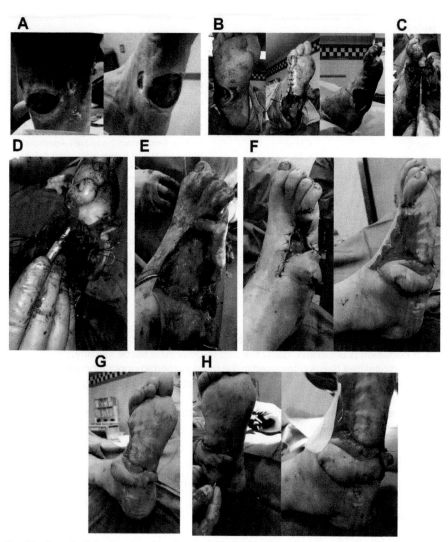

Fig. 10. Case 6, diabetic with chronic sub–fifth metatarsal base ulceration. (*A*) Chronic sub–fifth metatarsal ulcer. (*B*) Post-débridement and fifth ray disarticulation; note fifth digit fillet and delay. (*C*) Note the distal perforating branch. (*D*) Perforating flap clamped and Doppler examination completed to ensure antegrade flow through dorsal and plantar digital arteries to allow successful separation as 2 separate flaps. (*E*) The fillet flap was divided. The plantar half was divided and inset dorsally to cover fourth MTPJ. (*F*) Donor site after inset of the flap which temporized with integra graft for later skin grafting. (*G*) Flap inset to cover the plantar defect; the dorsal digital artery flap was elevated along with DMA to allow for a large fasciocutaneous flap to cover defect. (*H*) The digital fillet flap, prick test indicating intact arterial flow to the flap. Note pinpoint bleeding indicating intact arterial flow. (*Courtesy of* S. Masadeh, DPM, Cincinnati, OH.)

Table 2 Fillet flap classification as presented by Küntscher		
Type A	A1	Finger and toe flaps—pedicled
	A2	Island—isolated on neurovascular bundle
	A3	Microsurgical—free flap
Type B	B1	Limb flaps—pedicled
	B2	Island—isolated on neurovascular bundle
	B3	Microsurgical—free flap
Type C	C1	B1 flap from intact body area—pedicled
	C2	Island—isolated on neurovascular bundle
	C3	Microsurgical—free flap

Data from Kuntscher MV, Erdmann D, Homann HH, et al. The Concept of Fillet Flaps: Classification, Indications, and Analysis of Their Clinical Value. Plast Reconstr Surg. 2000;108(4):12.

coverage of a heel soft tissue deficit, their use has continued to expand to coverage of other areas of the foot and ankle and even as a free tissue transfer for hand reconstruction. This practice of spare parts surgery makes an effort to utilize soft tissue, that normally would be discarded, for soft tissue coverage.

CLINICS CARE POINTS

- The digital fillet flap offers a unique ability to cover deficits.
- If perfusion is uncertain, delay the flap to determine tissue viability.
- The digital fillet flap is often used in the multi-comorbid population who are prone to complications. The surgeon must anticipate and have resources available to manage complications.
- Spare parts surgery can avoid increased morbidity and should be considered after proper medical and surgical workup.

DISCLOSURE

No authors have relevant commercial or financial interests.

REFERENCES

1. Lavery LA, Armstrong DG, Wunderlich RP, et al. Diabetic foot syndrome: evaluating the prevalence and incidence of foot pathology in mexican americans and non-hispanic whites from a diabetes disease management cohort. Diabetes Care 2003;26:1435–8.
2. Moberg E. Evaluation and management of nerve injuries in the hand. Surg Clin North Am 1964;44:10.
3. Schade VL. Digital fillet flaps: a systematic review. Foot Ankle Spec 2014;8(4): 273–8.
4. Kelikian AS, Sarrafian SK. Sarrafian's anatomy of the foot and ankle: descriptive, topographic, functional. Philadelphia: Lippincott Williams & Wilkins; 2011.
5. DiLandro AC, Lilja EC, Lepore FL, et al. The prevalence of the arcuate artery a cadaveric study of 72 feet. JAPMA 2001;91(6):6.
6. Yamada T, Gloviczki P, Bower TC, et al. Variations of the arterial anatomy of the foot. Am J Surg 1993;166:6.

7. Snyder GB, Edgerton MT. The principle of the island neurovascular flap in the management of ulcerated anesthetic weightbearing areas of the lower extremity. Plast Reconstr Surg 1965;36(5):11.
8. Kaplan I. Neurovascular island flap in the treatment of trophic ulceration of the heel. Br J Plast Surg 1965;22(2):6.
9. Emmett AJJ. The filleted toe flap. Br J Plast Surg 1976;29:3.
10. Morain WD. Island toe flaps in neurotrophic ulcers of the foot and ankle. Ann Plast Surg 1984;13(1):8.
11. Lin CH, Wei FC, CHen HC. Filleted toe flap for chronic forefoot ulcer reconstruction. Ann Plast Surg 2000;44(4):5.
12. Küntscher MV, Erdmann D, Homann HH, et al. The concept of fillet flaps classification indications and analysis of their clinical value. Plast Reconstr Surg 2001; 108(4):12.
13. Kalbermatten DF, Kalbermatten NT, Haug M, et al. Use of a combined pedicled toe fillet flap. Scand J Plast Reconstr Surg Hand Surg 2004;38(5):301–5.
14. Yarmel D, Dormans JP, Pawel BR, et al. Recurrent pedal hobnail (Dabska-retiform) hemangioendothelioma with forefoot reconstructive surgery using a digital fillet flap. J Foot Ankle Surg 2008;47(5):487–93.
15. Aerden D, Vanmierlo B, Denecker N, et al. Primary closure with a filleted hallux flap after transmetatarsal amputation of the big toe for osteomyelitis in the diabetic foot: a short series of four cases. Int J Low Extrem Wounds 2012;11(2):80–4.
16. Eliezer S, Shai A, Yoav R, et al. Medial forefoot fillet flap for primary closure of transmetatarsal amputation: a series of four cases. Foot (Edinb) 2017;33:53–6.
17. Eneroth M, Apelqvist J, Stenstrom A. Clinical characteristics and outcome in 223 diabetic patients with deep foot infections. Foot Ankle Int 1997;18(11):6.
18. Pappalardo M, Laurence VG, Lin YT. Chimeric free vascularized metatarsophalangeal joint with toe fillet flap: a technique for reconstruction of the posttraumatic metacarpophalangeal joint with concomitant soft tissue defect. J Hand Surg Am 2018;43(2):193.e1-6.
19. Sun W, Chen C, Wang Z, et al. Full-length finger reconstruction for proximal amputation with expanded wraparound great toe flap and vascularized second toe joint. Ann Plast Surg 2016;77(5):539–46.
20. Shen XF, Mi JY, Xue MY, et al. Modified great toe wraparound flap with preservation of plantar triangular flap for reconstruction of degloving injuries of the thumb and fingers: long-term follow-up. Plast Reconstr Surg 2016;138(1):155–63.

Intrinsic Muscle Flaps for Coverage of Small Defects in the Foot

Grace Chuang Craig, DPM

KEYWORDS

- Muscle flap • Diabetic foot ulcer • Osteomyelitis • Limb salvage
- Extensor digitorum brevis • Abductor digiti minimi • Flexor hallucis brevis
- Abductor hallucis brevis

KEY POINTS

- Muscle flaps remain often the first choice when dealing with bone infections associated with osteomyelitis, soft tissue infections, and large cavities.
- The muscle obliterates dead spaces and enhances regenerative capacity at the defect.
- Distal forefoot defects are a challenge in the absence of microsurgical expertise. Intrinsic local flaps of the foot can be an option for defect coverage.

INTRODUCTION

Loss of soft tissue coverage distally around the foot poses threats of amputation of exposed boney structures. Exposure of critical structures such as joints, bones, ligaments, and tendons necessitates expeditious closure. The longer these structures remain open to the environment, the higher the risk is for that patient developing osteomyelitis and an amputation. An amputation of a portion of the foot leads to loss of the biomechanical structural integrity of the foot. This promulgates an imbalance with its inherent risks of developing new ulcers. This in turn potentiates the limb loss cycle.

Soft tissue reconstruction of the lower extremity often requires coverage by local or distant flaps. Using vascularized flaps to attain rapid wound closure diminishes the risk in immunocompromised patients. This not only allows for immediate closure but also has the ability to perfuse the area with parenteral antibiotics.

Muscle flaps remain often the first choice when dealing with bone infections associated with osteomyelitis, soft tissue infections, and large cavities by obliterating dead spaces and enhanced regenerative capacity at the defect.[1] Every muscle is a potential flap if the surgeon has the knowledge of its functional and vascular anatomy.[2] Major advantages of muscle flaps are reliable soft tissue coverage of bone and tendons

Elevate Foot and Ankle, 2880 Plymouth Avenue, Rocky River, OH 44116, USA
E-mail address: gracecraigdpm@gmail.com

Clin Podiatr Med Surg 37 (2020) 789–802
https://doi.org/10.1016/j.cpm.2020.07.006
0891-8422/20/© 2020 Elsevier Inc. All rights reserved.

podiatric.theclinics.com

and preservation of arteries of the lower extremity.[3–5] Because common local distally based muscle flaps have difficulty reaching the forefoot plantar region, these defects are normally treated by free tissue transfer.[6] However, free tissue transfer procedures are relatively complex, time consuming, and requires microsurgical expertise and donor-site morbidity, which may not be suitable to candidates who are high risk for long operating times and extensive anesthesia risk.[7,8] Therefore, distal forefoot defects are challenging in the absence of microsurgical expertise. Intrinsic local flaps of the foot can be an option.

Dissection of intrinsic muscle flaps are relatively straightforward. The donor site morbidity is minimal and most of the donor site can be closed primarily while the muscle is covered with either an allograft matrix or a split-thickness skin graft. The drawback of intrinsic muscle flaps is its limited bulk. The intrinsic muscles of the foot are all classified as Mathes and Nahai type II flap muscles with one dominant vascular pedicle and one or more distal minor pedicles.[2] Intrinsic muscle flaps includes extensor digitorum brevis (EDB) muscle, abductor digiti minimi (ADM) muscle, flexor hallucis brevis (FHB) muscle, abductor hallucis brevis (AHB) muscle, and flexor digitorum brevis (FDB) muscle. The intrinsic muscles of the foot's anatomy, vascular supply, and dissection techniques will be discussed to aid surgeons in reconstruction of the foot and ankle.

EXTENSOR DIGITORUM BREVIS MUSCLE FLAP

The EDB can be raised for a proximally based, medially based, and distally based flap. The EDB muscle can also be used as a free flap, a flow through flap, and a vascularized nerve graft when harvested with the deep peroneal nerve.[2,9,10] The EDB muscle can cover defects over the base of the toes, medial or lateral midfoot, and even as far proximally as the tibial tuberosity.[11]

Anatomy

The EDB originates from the lateral anterior superior aspect of the calcaneus in front of the groove for peroneus brevis in addition to the stem of inferior extensor retinaculum of the foot. The origin can vary frequently from adjacent bones and ligaments.[12] The EDB inserts with a distinct slip that runs distally, superficial to the dorsalis pedis artery and insert onto the base of the proximal phalanx of the great toe. The distinct slip is named extensor hallucis brevis. The other slips of the EDB attach to the lateral sides of the toe extensors and the proximal phalanx for the second, third, and fourth digits. The muscle belly is approximately 7 cm × 4 cm with a surface area of 30 cm and lies deep to the extensor digitorum longus (EDL) of the foot.[13]

There are anatomic variations and morphometry of the EDB. Additional bellies were observed for EDB and mostly occupied the position between first and second bellies of the EDB, inserting onto the fascia covering the dorsal interosseous muscle. Occasionally, the EDB may have 2 or 3 distinct heads and more rarely the whole muscle may be absent. An extra tendon may also join the long extensor tendon of the fifth digit.[14–17]

Vascular Supply

EDB receives its arterial supply from the lateral tarsal artery (LTA), which is a branch of the dorsalis pedis artery (DPA). There may be variations of the LTA with 2 LTA instead of one (**Fig. 1**). The LTA forms an arterial anastomosis with the branches of lateral plantar artery and perforating branch of the peroneal artery deep to the EDB muscle. The medial tarsal branch (MTA) from the medial plantar artery supplies the minor pedicle to the EDB.[12]

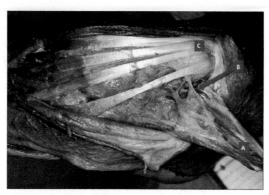

Fig. 1. (A) Extensor digitorum brevis muscle belly. (B) Lateral tarsal artery from the dorsalis pedis artery supplying the extensor digitorum brevis muscle. (C) Extensor digitorum longus tendons.

The EDB can be a medially based flap based on the medial tarsal branch. Distally based EDB flap is based on the communication between the DPA and the plantar arch at the level of the tarsometatarsal joint and another in the first web space with the first dorsal metatarsal artery (FDMA).[11]

Surgical Technique

Preoperatively, ultrasound Doppler is used to trace the course of the DPA to ensure there is retrograde flow in the DPA from the plantar arch after occluding the DPA proximally.

A curved incision is placed at the dorsal medial foot extending from the lateral malleolus to the first web space. EDB muscle is identified in the plane deeper to the EDL tendons. The EDL tendons are retracted laterally.

Distally based extensor digitorum brevis muscle flap

After dissecting the DPA along with the LTA supplying the EDB muscle, vascular clamps are applied to the MTA and DPA proximally to assess the retrograde perfusion of the EDB muscle flap before ligating the DPA proximally. The muscle is dissected from its origin from the sinus tarsi, keeping the LTA branches from the DPA intact. The branches of the superficial and deep peroneal nerve are identified and preserved to avoid muscle atrophy. The DPA is ligated proximally at the inferior edge of the extensor retinaculum and the MTA is ligated just distally. The DPA is dissected distally to the level of the communicating branch at the tarsometatarsal joint level. If the arch of rotation of the EDB muscle flap to the defect is adequate, dissection can be stopped. If not, the dissection is continued distally where the DPA continues into the FDMA. Victor and colleagues[18] ensure dissecting is used in the interosseous muscle along with the FDMA when the FDMA is intramuscular to ensure there is a cuff of muscle around the FDMA vessel to prevent vasospasm. There may be anatomic variations of the course of the FDMA superficial to the interosseous muscle or within the muscle. Dissection is continued till the communicating branch in the first web space. The flap is then advanced into the defect.

Proximally based extensor digitorum brevis flap

The extensor tendons are released just distally to the muscle bellies. The EDB is freed off the deep proximal attachment starting from the tarsal bones in the midfoot, to its origin in the calcaneus. The EDB is then dissected proximally with distal perforators ligated. The DPA is then ligated distal at the origin of the lateral tarsal artery, which will allow the EDB to have an extra arc of rotation (**Fig. 2**). To further increase the extension, the EDB can be dissected proximally with the extensor retinaculum divided.

ABDUCTOR DIGITI MINIMI MUSCLE FLAP

The ADM muscle can be used for small coverage of midfoot and hindfoot defects, including the calcaneus and lateral malleolus.

Anatomy

The ADM muscle is located in the first layer of the lateral foot between the flexor digitorum brevis medially and the fifth metatarsal and cuboid laterally. The ADM originates from the medial and lateral calcaneal tubercles, the plantar aponeurosis, and adjacent intermuscular septum. The muscle inserts onto the lateral aspect of the base of the fifth proximal phalanx of the fifth digit.[19]

Vascular Supply

ADM muscle is supplied by the lateral plantar artery. Specifically, the main vascular supply is the proximal branch of the lateral plantar artery, which is located approximately 1 to 2 cm proximally from the styloid process of the fifth metatarsal bone.[20]

Surgical Technique

The incision is made along the fifth metatarsal bone. Dissection is then performed at the insertion site of the ADM muscle at the lateral base of the fifth digit proximal phalanx. The tendon is then transected at its insertion. Dissection is performed from distal to proximal. The ADM muscle is then free from the flexor digiti minimi brevis muscle with blunt dissection. During the dissection, several minor pedicles are encountered and ligated. Dissection is stopped approximately 1 to 2 cm proximal from the styloid process of the fifth metatarsal to avoid injury to the major pedicle (**Fig. 3**). The nerve to the muscle should also be preserved to minimize muscle atrophy, which also passes along with the artery. If the arc of the muscle rotation is further needed, freeing the muscle from its insertion may be needed. The muscle flap is carefully rotated into the defect (**Fig. 4**).

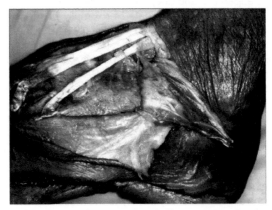

Fig. 2. Proximally based extensor digitorum brevis flap covering the sinus tarsi defect.

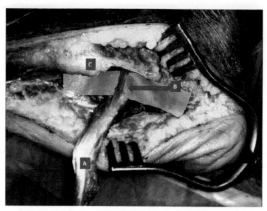

Fig. 3. (A) Abductor digiti minimi muscle belly. (B) Proximal branch of the lateral plantar artery supplying the abductor digiti minimi muscle. (C) Styloid process of the fifth metatarsal bone.

FLEXOR HALLUCIS BREVIS MUSCLE FLAP

The FHB muscle can cover deficits over the first metatarsophalangeal joint.[21]

Anatomy

The lateral head of the FHB muscle originates from the medial part of the plantar surface of the cuboid, posterior to the groove for the peroneus longus tendon and from the adjacent part of the lateral cuneiform. The medial head of the FHB muscle originates from the deep attachment that is continuous with the lateral division of the tibialis posterior tendon and a more superficial attachment to the middle band of the medial intermuscular septum of the foot. The muscle inserts with one portion into either side of the base of the proximal phalanx of the hallux and both sesamoids. The other portion blends with the abductor hallucis and the adductor hallucis.

Vascular

The FHB is supplied from the medial plantar artery and the metatarsal branches of the plantar arch (**Fig. 5**).

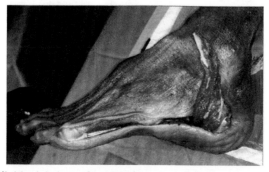

Fig. 4. Abductor digiti minimi muscle rotated to cover defect.

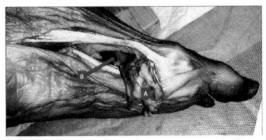

Fig. 5. (A) Flexor hallucis brevis muscle. (B) Metatarsal branch of the plantar arch supplying the flexor hallucis brevis muscle.

Surgical Technique

The incision is made along the glabrous junction of the medial aspect of the foot. Dissection is performed, dissection plantar lateral from the AHB tendon (**Fig. 6**). Blunt dissection is performed by separating the FHB from the AHB tendon. Both heads of the FHB are separated from their origin and reflected distally after the neurovascular supply is severed from the medial plantar nerve and vessels. The muscle is then reflected over the deficit (**Fig. 7**).

ABDUCTOR HALLUCIS MUSCLE FLAP

The abductor hallucis (ABH) muscle is usually used as a proximally based flap to cover defects at the medial aspect of the foot. In this fashion it can also cover defects of the heel as a turnover island flap based on a single supplying vascular branch from the medial plantar artery (MPA). The muscle can also be used as a distally based muscle flap to cover forefoot deficits.

The ABH muscle has a small muscle bulk, which may not be adequate for coverage of large wounds. A study by Attinger and colleagues[9] reported that ABH muscle flaps are ideal for closure of defects less than or equal to 3×6 cm^2 at the foot or ankle with exposed bone, joint, or tendon.

Anatomy

The ABH muscle is the most superficial muscle in the medial compartment of the first layer of the plantar foot. The muscle originates predominantly from the flexor

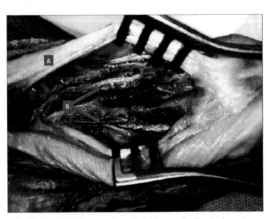

Fig. 6. (A) Abductor hallucis muscle tendon. (B) Flexor hallucis brevis muscle bellies.

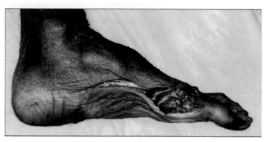

Fig. 7. Flexor hallucis brevis muscle rotated to cover the first metatarsal head deficit.

retinaculum and posterior calcaneal tuberosity. There are a few fibers of ABH that originates from the intermuscular septum and the FHB.[22] The muscle inserts distally at the base of the proximal phalanx of the hallux and the tibial sesamoid.

Vascular Supply

AHB flap receives its blood supply from minor and major pedicles in a retrograde fashion from both the dorsal arterial network and the deep plantar system through communicating branches with the MPA. Because the proposed flap has a double source of vascularity, the presence of a single, patent dorsalis pedis or tibial artery alone would suffice for using the flap with safety. Because the lateral plantar artery is not sacrificed during flap dissection, the vascularity of the sole and the entire foot is preserved.

Surgical Technique

Distally based abductor hallucis brevis muscle flap
A skin incision is made along the glabrous junction of the medial aspect of the foot. Dissection is deepened through the subcutaneous layer, and care is taken to identify and ligate the medial venous plexus when encountered. The abductor hallucis tendon is identified distally, and a vessel loupe is inserted around it for manipulation (see **Fig. 6**). The abductor hallucis muscle is dissected out proximally. Minor perforator arteries can be identified in-between the ABH and the FHB muscle belly. AHB muscle is then skeletonized from the FHB tendon using blunt dissection. A handheld intraoperative Doppler is then used to identify a brisk signal from the minor pedicles. A vascular clamp was then applied to the proximal pedicle. The muscle cut was evaluated for bleeding based on the distal pedicle. This intraoperatively confirms adequate vascularity to the muscle flap. The proximal minor pedicle is then ligated, and the muscle is turned down distally to cover the deficit. To increase the arc of rotation for distally based flap, the lateral plantar artery may be cut and sacrificed when there's sufficient blood supply by the DPA.

Proximally based abductor hallucis brevis muscle flap
The insertion of the tendon is isolated, transected, and reflected proximally. Multiple perforating branches of the medial plantar artery are identified and ligated to allow further proximal reflection and rotation of the muscle belly into the defect. The last perforating branch of the medial plantar artery is encountered approximately 0.5 to 1 cm distal to the navicular tuberosity (**Fig. 8**). Sacrificing the last perforator may be needed to increase the range of the muscle rotation for more proximal defects. The muscle belly is then carefully reflected and rotated into the defect.

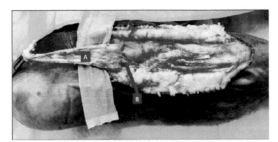

Fig. 8. (A) Abductor hallucis muscle belly. (B) A pedicle supplying the abductor hallucis muscle. (*Courtesy of* S. Masadeh, DPM, Cincinnati, OH.)

FLEXOR DIGITORUM BREVIS MUSCLE FLAP

FDB muscle flap can be used to cover the posterior heel, lower Achilles tendon, or medial or lateral malleoli. The muscle is easy to separate without affecting the vascularity of the foot. Some limitations of flexor digitorum brevis muscle flap include extensive skin defects that involve the instep area as well as areas that are beyond the

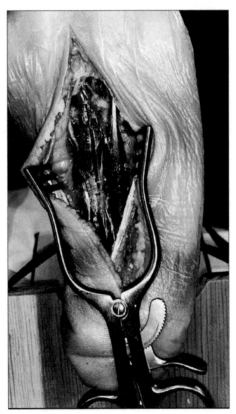

Fig. 9. Flexor digitorum brevis muscle with its tendons. The plantar fascia is incised and retracted.

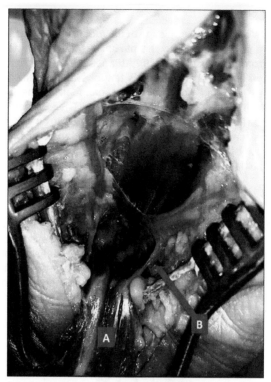

Fig. 10. (A) Flexor digitorum brevis muscle belly. (B) Lateral plantar artery pedicle supplying the flexor digitorum brevis muscle.

instep area. Because the FDB muscle flap is limited in bulk and reach, it may not fill the entire defect.[9]

Anatomy

The FDB muscle lies immediately deep to the central part of the plantar aponeurosis. The muscle originates from the central part of the plantar aponeurosis, medial tubercle of calcaneal tuberosity, and from the medial and lateral intermuscular septa. The FDB divides into 4 tendons for third, fourth, and fifth digits. Each tendon is divided into 2 slips at the base of their proximal phalanges and attaches to both sides of the shaft of the middle phalanx. The FDB is bordered by the ABH muscle medially and the ADM laterally.

The most common variation of FDB is absence of tendon to the fifth digit with the tendon arising as a separate muscle. The incidence of absence of flexor digitorum brevis slip to the fifth digit is reported as 21%, 100%, 63%, and 18% among different researches.[23–26]

Vascular

The major blood supply to the FDB is the lateral plantar artery (LPA) pedicle supplying the muscle at the proximal third of the muscle belly. There are also minor pedicles from the LPA distally and small pedicles from the medial plantar artery.

Surgical Technique

The incision is made on the plantar midline of the foot from the calcaneus to the meta-tarsal pad. Incision is made deep to the plantar fascia where the plantar fascia is bluntly dissected from the muscle (**Fig. 9**). At times the plantar fascia is left with the muscle flap to augment its bulk. The FDB tendons are identified and transected. The muscle is then reflected proximally, dissecting off of the quadratus plantae without severing the medial or lateral plantar arteries. The LPA perforators are identified during dissection (**Fig. 10**). The muscle is then rotated to cover the defect (**Fig. 11**). If the arc of rotation needed to be increased, the LPA can be divided and elevated in the midplantar aspect of the foot with the flap to cover the posterior heel, lower Achilles tendon, or medial/lateral malleoli.[27]

POSTOPERATIVE CARE

Postoperative management after definitive coverage with intrinsic muscle flap, the patients are followed in the outpatient setting every 10 to 14 days for clinical evaluation and serial radiographs if needed. When standard bolster dressings are used, they are left in place for 2 to 3 weeks, depending on the clinical presentation at the first postoperative visit. The bolster is removed at the first postoperative visit only if it is macerated or malodorous; otherwise, it is left in place for approximately 2 to 3 weeks. If

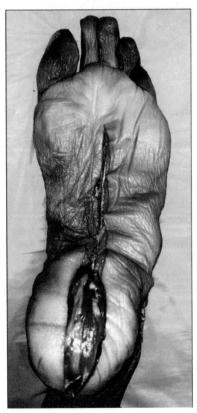

Fig. 11. Flexor digitorum brevis muscle rotated to cover the heel deficit.

negative pressure wound therapy is used as the bolster dressing, it is left in place and untouched for about 4 to 5 days following surgery, and it is then replaced with a moist to dry dressing.

Immobilization is requisite, whether through external fixation, casting, or splinting until satisfactory and stable coverage of the muscle has been established. The patients' weight-bearing and immobilization status depends on the corresponding osseous and soft-tissue procedures performed. If a drain is placed as prophylaxis against hematoma formation, it is removed approximately 2 to 3 days after surgery.

DISCUSSION

Intrinsic muscle flap is easy to harvest, reliable, durable, and a quick option to reconstruct ulcers of the forefoot, midfoot, and hindfoot. Reconstruction of weight-bearing areas are difficult to resurface due to its unique anatomy, but by using intrinsic muscle flaps, it can provide a well-padded tissue for durable and biomechanically proper reconstruction.[28]

When choosing the appropriate reconstructive option for the treatment of deficits or ulcers, the dimensions and anatomic location need to be assessed. It is also important to evaluate that the muscles have adequate blood supply in order to achieve successful results.

Unfortunately, complications can occur with intrinsic muscle flaps. Postoperatively, partial flap loss has been observed. Patients can also develop seroma and hematoma at the donor site, which may require surgical drainage.[29]

The intrinsic muscle flaps for treatment of deficits of the foot have provided surgeons a safe, effective, viable, and reliable one-stage reconstruction procedure.

CLINICAL CARE POINTS

Extensor Digitorum Brevis Muscle Flap
- The muscle can be raised for a proximally based, medially based, and distally based flap to cover defects over the base of the toes, medial or lateral midfoot, and even as far proximally as the tibial tuberosity.
- The muscle belly is approximately 7 cm × 4 cm with a surface area of 30 cm.
- EDB receives its arterial supply from the lateral tarsal artery (LTA) where there may be 2 LTA instead of one.
- The MTA from the medial plantar artery supplies the minor pedicle to the EDB.
- The EDB can be a medially based flap based on the medial tarsal branch. Distally based EDB flap is based on the communication between the DPA and the plantar arch at the level of the tarsometatarsal joint and another in the first web space with the FDMA.
- Preoperatively, ultrasound Doppler is used to trace the course of the DPA to ensure there is retrograde flow in the DPA from the plantar arch after occluding the DPA proximally.
- To increase the arc of rotation for distally based flaps, dissection is continued distally where the DPA continues into the FDMA, ensuring FDMA is intramuscular with a cuff of muscle around the FDMA vessel to prevent vasospasm.
- For a proximally based flap, the DPA is ligated distally at the origin of the lateral tarsal artery, which will allow the EDB to have an extra arc of rotation.

Abductor Digiti Minimi Muscle Flap
- The muscle can be used for small coverage of midfoot and hindfoot defects, including the calcaneus and lateral malleolus.

- The main vascular supply is the proximal branch of the lateral plantar artery, which is located approximately 1 to 2 cm proximally from the styloid process of the fifth metatarsal bone.
- Dissection is stopped approximately 1 to 2 cm proximal from the styloid process of the fifth metatarsal to avoid injury to the major pedicle.
- The nerve to the muscle should be preserved to minimize muscle atrophy, which passes along with the artery.
- If the arc of the muscle rotation is further needed, freeing the muscle from its insertion may be needed.

FHB Muscle Flap

- The muscle can cover deficits over the first metatarsophalangeal joint.
- Both heads of the FHB are separated from their origin and reflected distally after the neurovascular supply is severed from the medial plantar nerve and vessels.

Abductor Hallucis Muscle Flap

- The muscle has a small muscle bulk and is ideal for closure of defects less than or equal to 3×6 cm^2
- With a double source of vascularity, the presence of a single, patent dorsalis pedis or tibial artery alone would suffice for using the flap with safety.
- To increase the arc of rotation for distally based flap, the lateral plantar artery may be cut and sacrificed when there's sufficient blood supply by the dorsalis pedis artery.
- The last perforating branch of the medial plantar artery is encountered approximately 0.5 to 1 cm distal to the navicular tuberosity. Sacrificing the last perforator may be needed to increase the range of the muscle rotation for more proximal defects.

Flexor Digitorum Brevis Muscle Flap

- Limitations of flexor digitorum brevis muscle flap includes extensive skin defects that involve the instep area as well as areas that are beyond the instep area because FDB is limited in bulk and reach.
- The most common variation of FDB is absence of tendon to the fifth digit with the tendon arising as a separate muscle. The incidence of absence of flexor digitorum brevis slip to the fifth digit is reported as 21%, 100%, 63%, and 18% among different researches.
- The major blood supply to the FDB is the lateral plantar artery (LPA) pedicle supplying the muscle at the proximal third of the muscle belly. There are also minor pedicles from the LPA distally and small pedicles from the medial plantar artery.
- At times the plantar fascia is left with the muscle flap to augment its bulk.
- If the arc of rotation needed to be increased, the LPA can be divided and elevated in the midplantar aspect of the foot with the flap to cover the posterior heel, lower Achilles tendon, or medial/lateral malleoli.

DISCLOSURE

The author has nothing to disclose.

REFERENCES

1. Ger R. The operative treatment of the advanced stasis ulcer: a preliminary communication. Am Surg 1966;111:659–63.
2. Ger R. The management of chronic ulcers of the dorsum of the foot by muscle transposition and free skin grafting. Br J Plast Surg 1996;29:199–204.

3. Ger R, Schessel E. Prevention of major amputations in non-ischemic lower limb lesions. J Am Coll Surg 2005;201:898–905.

4. Ger R. The management of pre-tibial skin loss. Surgery 1968;63:757–63.

5. Ger R. Operative treatment of the advanced stasis ulcer using muscle transposition: a follow-up study. Am J Surg 1970;120:376–80.

6. Ger R. The techniques of muscle transposition in the operative treatment of traumatic and ulcerative lesions of the leg. J Trauma 1971;11:502–10.

7. Ger R. The surgical management of ulcers of the heel. Surg Gynecol Obstet 1975;140:909–91.

8. Mathes SJ, Nahal F. Clinical atlas of muscle and musculocutaneous flaps. St Louis (MO): C. V. Mosby Company; 1979.

9. Attinger CE, Ducic I, Cooper P, et al. The role of intrinsic muscle flaps of the foot for bone coverage in foot and ankle defects in diabetic and nondiabetic patients. Plast Reconstr Surg 2002;110:1047–54.

10. Landi A, Soragni O, Monteleone M. The extensor digitorum brevis muscle island flap for soft tissue loss around ankle. Plast Reconstr Surg 1985;75:892–897.21.

11. Bakhach J, Demiri E, Chahidi N, et al. Extensor digitorum brevis muscle flap: new refinements. Plast Reconstr Surg 1998;102:103–10.

12. Swathi, Geetha GN, Athavale S, et al. Morphology and neurovascular supply of extensor digitorum brevis muscle of the foot in humans: implications for reconstructive surgeries. Indian J Clin Anat Physiol 2017;4(1):106–11.

13. Sirasanagandlav S, Swamy R, Nayak SB, et al. Analysis of the morphometry and variations in the extensor digitorum brevis muscle: an anatomic guide for muscle flap and tendon transfer surgical dissection. Anat Cell Biol 2013;46(3):198–202.

14. Bergman RA, Afifi AK, Miyauchi R. Extensor Digitorum Brevis (Pedis). Illustrated encyclopedia of human anatomic variation: Opus I: Muscular system: alphabetical listing of muscles: E. Anatomy Atlases. [cited 2013 Sep 1].

15. Anson BJ. Morris' human anatomy. 12th edition. New York: McGrawHill Book Co.; 1966.

16. Henle J. Handbuch der Muskellehre des Menschen. In: Handbuch der systematischen Anatomie des Menschen. Braunschweig (Germany): Verlag von Friedrich Vieweg und Sohn; 1871.

17. Macalister A. Additional observation on muscular anomalies in human anatomy (third series), with a catalogue of the principal muscular variations hitherto published. Trans R Ir Acad 1875;25:1–134.

18. Victor J, J V, PP L, et al. The distally based extensor digitorum brevis muscle flap in resurfacing distal foot defects. International Journal of Current Medical And Applied Sciences 2018;21(1):14–7.

19. Yoshimora Y, Nakajima T, Kami T. Distally based abductor digiti minimi flap. Ann Plast Surg 1985;14(4):375–7.

20. Ger R. Abductor digiti minimi muscle flap. In: Strauch B, Vasconez LO, Hall Findlay EJ, editors. Grabb's encyclopedia of flaps, vol. 3. Boston: Little, Brown; 1990. p. 1663–5.

21. Mahan KT, Feehery RV. Flexor hallucis brevis muscle flap. J Foot Surg 1991;30(3):284–8.

22. Chittoria RK, Pratap H, Yekappa HS. Abductor hallucis: anatomical variation and its clinical implications in the reconstruction of chronic nonhealing ulcers and defects of foot. Adv Wound Care (New Rochelle) 2015;4(12):719–23.

23. Bergman RA, Thompson SA, Afifi AK, et al. Compendium of human anatomic variations. Baltimore: Urban and Schwarzenberg; 1988.

24. Lobo SW, Menezes RG, Mamata S, et al. Phylogenetic variation in flexor digitorum brevis: a Nepalese cadaveric study. Nepal Med Coll J 2008;10:230–2.
25. Nathan H, Globe H. Flexor digitorum brevis – anatomical variations. Anat Anz 1974;135:295–301.
26. Yalçin B, Ozan H. Some variations of the musculus flexor digitorum brevis. Anat Sci Int 2005;80:189–92.
27. Hartrampf CR, Scheflan M, Bostwick J. The flexor digitorum brevis muscle island pedicle flap: a new dimension in heel reconstruction. Plast Reconstr Surg 1980; 66(2):264–70.
28. Sakai N, Yoshida T, Okumura H. Distal plantar area reconstruction using a flexor digitorum brevis muscle flap with reverse-flow lateral plantar artery. Br J Plast Surg 2001;54(2):170–3.
29. Ortak T, Ozdemir R, Ulusoy MG, et al. Reconstruction of heel defects with a proximally based abductor hallucis muscle flap. J Foot Ankle Surg 2005;44(4): 265–70.

Orthobiologics and Skin Grafting

The Role of Dermal Regenerative Templates in Complex Lower Extremity Wounds

Jordan A. Henning, DPM[a,1], Michael D. Liette, DPM[b],
Mohamed Laklouk, MD[c], Mohamed Fadel, MD[d,2],
Suhail Masadeh, DPM[e,*]

KEYWORDS

- Matrix • Lower extremity • Limb salvage • Wound care • Synthetic graft
- Orthobiologics

KEY POINTS

- Dermal regenerative templates (DRTs) are composed of a bilayer that minimizes fluid loss and bacterial invasion while recreating a dermal layer.
- DRTs serve as a scaffold that promotes host cells infiltration.
- DRTs create a vascularized wound bed capable of accepting a skin graft.
- DRTs' successful incorporation and dermal regeneration are highly dependent on wound bed preparation.
- DRTs have shown efficacy in reducing contractures.

INTRODUCTION

The management of complex wounds of the lower extremity is challenging, particularly in the presence of exposed bone, tendon, or joint capsule. These structures when exposed are prone to desiccation, chronic inflammation, and necrosis. Furthermore, their wound beds have poor vascularity, rendering them incapable of supporting a skin graft.[1] Surgeons often rely on the plastic reconstructive ladder to decide on the appropriate surgical modality for these defects. The reconstructive ladder offers a stepwise approach for the management of soft tissue defects and is presented in

[a] University of Cincinnati Medical Center, Cincinnati Veterans Affairs Medical Center, Cincinnati, OH, USA; [b] University of Cincinnati Medical Center, 231 Albert Sabin Way, ML 0513, Cincinnati, OH 45276, USA; [c] Faculty of Medicine, Minia University, Doctors Building Minia University Second Floor, 10th Ramadan Street, Minia, Egypt; [d] Orthopedic and Trauma Surgery, Minia University Hospital, Minia, Egypt; [e] University of Cincinnati Medical Center, Cincinnati Veteran Affairs Medical Center, 231 Albert Sabin Way, ML 0513, Cincinnati, OH 45276, USA
[1] Present address: 580 Walnut Street, Apartment 803, Cincinnati, OH 45202.
[2] Present address: Limb Reconstructive Surgery Center, 53 Nasr City, Cairo 11471, Egypt.
* Corresponding author.
E-mail address: masadesb@uc.edu

Clin Podiatr Med Surg 37 (2020) 803–820
https://doi.org/10.1016/j.cpm.2020.07.010
0891-8422/20/Published by Elsevier Inc.

Box 1.[2–5] The procedure selections change from simple to increasingly more complex as with progression up the ladder. With an increase in complexity there is an associated increase in morbidity.[2–5] In the clinical scenario of exposed critical structures, the ladder typically leads to the utilization of local or free flaps. The benefit of flap surgery is the transfer of vascularized tissue to these relatively avascular wounds to achieve healing. This type of reconstruction is extensive, however, requiring specialized surgical skills and facilities.[6] The ladder provides an excellent conceptual framework to address difficult wounds but is not without limitation. These limitations have been recognized and multiple modifications have been created that are beyond the scope of this article.[2–5,7] Despite these modifications, the reconstructive ladder overlooks major advancements in wound healing modalities.

Advancements in technological innovation and regenerative medicine have improved the ability to achieve durable closure in a variety of complex wounds. One such advancement is the use of dermal matrices, originally developed for burn reconstruction.[8–11] These dermal regenerative templates (DRTs) often are synthetic bilayers made up of an inner collagen and outer silicone layer.[9–13] The silicone layer functions similarly to the keratinized epidermis, providing a barrier to infection from environmental pathogens and regulating fluid loss.[9–13] The inner layer is an acellular bioactive matrix with comparable properties to the native dermal matrix.[9–13] This layer provides the framework to support revascularization, cell repopulation, and tissue remodeling.[9–13] The framework has a specific pore size of 70 μm to 200 μm, which allows the migration of the host fibroblasts and endothelial cells to form a vascularized neodermis.[9–11,14] Therefore, the use of DRTs leads to the formation of a vascularized wound bed, or neodermis, capable of supporting a split-thickness skin graft.[9–13] To understand the role and function of DRTs, a brief overview of the skin structure and phases of wound healing is presented.

SKIN STRUCTURE AND FUNCTION

The skin is the largest organ of the body and is composed of 2 distinct histologic layers with several physiologic and mechanical roles.[15,16] It serves to function as a barrier between the internal and the external environment and regulates fluid and temperature hemostasis, while also providing sensory feedback from various stimuli.[15,16] Knowledge of the structure, function, and repair mechanism of the integument is central

---

Box 1
Reconstructive ladder in the management of soft tissue deficits

Free flaps

Pedicled flaps

Local flaps

Tissue expansion

Full-thickness skin grafts

Split-thickness skin grafts

Delayed primary closure

Primary closure

Healing by secondary intention

for wound management. The skin is composed of 2 layers, the epidermis and the dermis, as seen in **Fig. 1**.[15,16] The epidermis is the outer layer, which is divided into multiple strata of cells. The thickness of the epidermis is variable based on anatomic location, with the palmer and plantar skin the thickest.[15,17] The most common type of cell in the epidermis is the keratinocyte, which forms in the deepest layer of the epidermis, the basal layer.[15,16,18] The basal layer is attached to the basement membrane by hemidesmosomes, which anchor the epidermis to the dermis, and contain melanocytes, Merkel cells, and Langerhans cells, additionally seen in **Fig. 1**.[16,19–21] The basal layer is mitotically active, continuously forming new keratinocytes to replace the outermost layer of the epidermis.[15,16,19] The keratinocytes migrate longitudinally, away from the dermal blood supply and toward the stratum corneum, undergoing terminal differentiation, otherwise known as keratinization.[19] As the keratinocytes reach the outer layer, they undergo apoptosis as well as hardening and flattening due to external pressures.[19] Excreted lipids (dehydrocholesterol) from Odland bodies within the keratinocytes in the stratum granulosum create cohesiveness and the hydrophobic properties of the skin.[16] Epidermal loss leads to the production of epidermal growth factors, signaling an increase in the mitotic activity of the basal keratinocytes, allowing for constant regeneration.[19] The epidermis is avascular and relies on the dermis for nutrition and waste removal via diffusion.[16]

The dermis is a moderately dense connective tissue composed of a papillary and a reticular layer.[15,16] It serves as a strong structural support and provides elasticity to the skin due to the presence of both collagen and elastin fibers.[15,16,19] The more

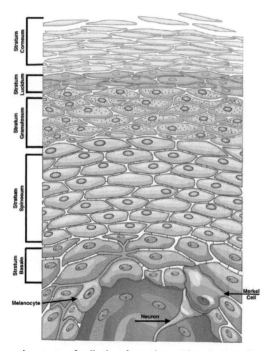

Fig. 1. Visualized are the strata of cells that form the epidermis. Traveling from superficial to deep, the layers are presented as stratum corneum, stratum lucidum, stratum granulosum, stratum spinosum, and the stratum basale. (*Courtesy of* S. Masadeh, DPM, Cincinnati, OH.)

superficial papillary dermis interdigitates with the epidermis via thin fibers of collagen to form the dermal-epidermal junction.[15,16] This upper layer of the dermis contains nerve endings, blood vessels, and lymphatic vessels, which provide the sensory feedback, nutrition, and waste disposal of the avascular epidermis, as demonstrated in **Fig. 2**.[15,16,19] The energy for mitosis and differentiation of keratinocytes is sustained by the diffusion of nutrients from the capillary network in the papillary dermis.[15] The deeper reticular dermis is composed of thick interconnected collagen strands, which provide strong structural support as well as elastic fibers for pliability.[15] The space between the elastic and collagen fibers is filled with a gel-like glycosaminoglycans matrix, creating a stable 3-dimensional construct.[15] This matrix contains fibroblasts, mast cells, and macrophages, the main cells required for wound healing and immune function.[15,16] Deep to the dermis is the subcutaneous layer, or the hypodermis, composed of adipocytes, which serve to insulate and redistribute pressure.[15,16] The epidermis and dermis can regenerate, whereas the epidermal appendages and subcutaneous tissue heal by scar formation.[19,22]

PHASES OF WOUND HEALING

Cells are divided into 3 groups based on their proliferative capability: labile, quiescent, and permanent.[23] Labile cells are continuously dividing, quiescent cells have a low proliferative ability requiring a stimulus to re-enter enter the cell cycle, and permanent

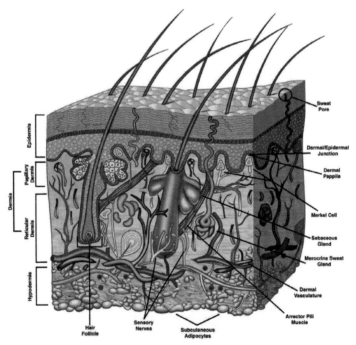

Fig. 2. The integument is separated into epidermal and dermal layers with the hypodermis, or subcutaneous layer, lying beneath. The dermis contains many appendages to support the epidermis, including sensory feedback, nutrition, and waste disposal. These functions are performed by the various appendages and vasculature within the dermal layers. (*Courtesy of* S. Masadeh, DPM, Cincinnati, OH.)

cells have left the cell cycle without an ability to further proliferate.[23] A wound represents a disruption in the normal structure and function of the skin and the underlying soft tissues. Wound healing is the body's response to an injury and an attempt to restore normal structure and function, involving 2 distinct processes, regeneration and repair. Wound regeneration occurs by the proliferation of the parenchyma and complete restoration of damaged cells.[22,23] Wound repair conversely occurs by proliferation of the tissue stroma resulting in granulation tissue.[22,23] Unlike regeneration, wound repair results in healing by fibrosis and scar formation; these processes are visualized in **Fig. 3**.[22,23]

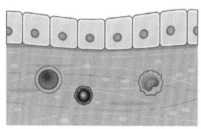

Intact integument

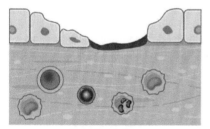

Superficial injury

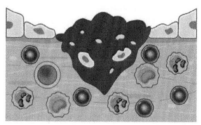

Deep injury

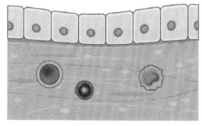

Regeneration

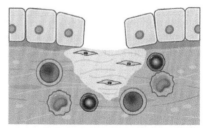

Repair with scar formation

Fig. 3. The type of healing that occurs after injury is divided into regeneration or repair/scar formation based on the extent of the injury. Superficial injuries heal with regeneration of the damaged tissues and deeper injuries rely on repair or scar formation to fill the deeper voids created. (*Courtesy of* S. Masadeh, DPM, Cincinnati, OH.)

Damage to the skin triggers an inflammatory cascade that activates the cells of wound healing.[23–26] These cellular events occur in 4 distinct yet overlapping phases.[23–26] These phases achieve wound healing by 3 mechanisms: filling the wound with connective tissue (granulation tissue) to restore the volume loss, stimulating contraction to reduce the width, and finally resurfacing of the wound by epithelialization.[27] Whether all 3 components are needed depends on the type and nature of the wound, as seen in **Fig. 3**. To understand the process of deposition, contraction, and epithelialization, the phases of wound healing are discussed.

INFLAMMATION

Inflammation is the process of specific vascular and cellular events that is intended to promote the removal of cellular debris and infectious organisms and initiate the repair process.[23,27] Bacteria release endotoxins that damage the adjacent tissue, leading to the activation of mast cells, which in turn produce histamine, leukotrienes, and prostaglandins.[23,27] These molecules bind to the receptors on endothelial vessels, promoting vasodilation and the formation of small gaps within the vessel walls. In addition to creating increased permeability, these molecules stimulate the endothelial cells to express P-selectin, allowing for the adhesion of phagocytic cells, such as neutrophils and monocytes.[23] During this process, these cells roll across the wall of the vessel, otherwise known as margination.[23] The monocyte or neutrophil then interacts with the P-CAMs receptor on the side of the endothelial cells, allowing them to squeeze through the newly created gaps in the capillary wall and into the interstitial space through a process known as diapedesis.[23] Once in the interstitial space, the phagocytic cell follow the chemical trail molecules to the site of injury, in a process called positive chemotaxis.[23,28] Upon encountering bacteria, monocytes synthesize and secrete interleukin (IL)-1 and tumor necrosis factor (TNF)-α, and neutrophils synthesize IL-8.[23,28] These chemokines stimulate the endothelial cells in the capillary wall to express E-selectins, I-CAMs and V-CAMs, recruiting additional cells to undergo diapedesis and migrate to the site of injury.[23,29]

INFLAMMATION (VASCULAR)

The inflammatory, or vascular phase, is defined as the vascular response of inflammation and is composed of 2 major processes: the development of a fibrin clot and pursuant coagulation to achieve hemostasis.[23] When the parenchymal and stromal cells are injured, bleeding occurs and the disrupted cellular membranes release chemical mediators of inflammation.[23] Blood vessel disruption activates the circulating platelets, allowing them to adhere and aggregate to form a fibrin clot.[23,27] The activated platelets and the mast cells within the injured site release chemokines and growth factors that promote migration and infiltration of leukocytes (neutrophils and monocytes) into the wounded area.[23,27] The formed fibrin clot serves as a scaffold matrix for the migrating leukocytes.[23,27]

INFLAMMATION (CELLULAR)

The cellular phase of inflammation begins at approximately 24 hours and continues for approximately 2 weeks.[26,27] Chemotactic factors generated through the coagulation phase recruit neutrophils and monocytes.[23,27,28] Initially, neutrophils are the first responders to kill and phagocytose bacteria as well as remove damaged matrix proteins.[23,26] Neutrophils release cytokines and recruit monocytes from circulation.[23,26] Once the monocytes enter the injured tissue, they differentiate into macrophages replacing the role of neutrophils.[23,26] Persistent wound contamination, however, pro-longs the presence of neutrophils and delays the progression of healing.[23] Chemotaxis is encouraged with the release of histamine and prostaglandins from mast cells, pro-moting vasodilation and increased capillary permeability.[23,27,28] The phagocytic cells release reactive oxygen species and other proteases to assist in clearing necrotic debris or damaged matrix structural components.[23,27] They also simultaneously pro-duce cytokines, such as fibroblast growth factor and epidermal growth factor, used to stimulate angiogenesis and recruit fibroblasts and epithelial cells as well as progres-sion into the proliferative phase.[24,26,28] The growth factors associated with the regen-erative or repair process are summarized in **Table 1**.

PROLIFERATIVE

The proliferative phase begins near day 3 and continues until approximately 21 days.[24,25,27] This phase has significant overlap with the others as the predominate cells are recruited early during the inflammatory phase and work simultaneously with the phagocytic cells to form granulation tissue.[24,25,27] It is during this time that robust angiogenesis occurs, granulation tissue is formed, collagen is deposited, and eventual epithelialization begins.[24,27] This leads to an increased delivery of the necessary growth factors and reagents for continued wound healing. Simultaneously, fibroblasts begin producing type III collagen and a glycosaminoglycan network to continue to fill the wound site with granulation tissue.[24,25,30] This stabilizes the newly formed vascu-lature network and creates a framework for the migrating epithelial cells.[24,25,30]

Table 1
Growth factors of the reparative or regenerative process of wound healing, their sources, and their primary functions

Growth Factor	Principle Sources	Function/Role
Platelet-derived growth factor	Platelets, macrophages, endothelial cells, keratinocytes, neutrophils	• ↑ Proliferation of smooth muscle cells and fibroblasts • ↑ Chemotaxis • ↑ Collagen synthesis • ↑ Macrophage activation • ↑ Mitogenesis
Fibroblast growth factor	Macrophages, mast cells, endothelial cells	• ↑ Proliferation of endothelial cells, keratinocytes, and fibroblasts • ↑ Collagen and elastin • ↑ Chemotaxis
TFG-β	Platelets, macrophages, endothelial cells, keratinocytes, fibroblasts	• ↑ ECM and fibroblasts • ↓ Proliferation of keratinocytes, endothelial cells • Chemotaxis
Vascular endothelial growth factor	Mesenchymal cells	• ↑ Vasculogenesis/sngiogenesis • Chemotaxis • ↑ Vessel permeability • ↑ Macrophage recruitment
Keratinocyte growth factor	Fibroblasts	• ↑ Keratinocyte migration, proliferation, and differentiation
Epidermal growth factor	Macrophages, keratinocytes	• ↑ Proliferation of keratinocytes, fibroblasts, endothelial cells • ↑ Keratinocyte migration

Fibroblasts within the granulation tissue are activated and acquire alpha-smooth muscle actin expression, becoming myofibroblasts.[31,32] The myofibroblasts continue to deposit extracellular matrix and assist in contraction of the wound.[31,32]

MATRIX REMODELING/SCAR FORMATION

During the final phase, the wound continues to remodel the newly formed extracellular matrix and cross-links the previously deposited collagen fibers. Myofibroblasts continue to contract the wound to decrease the surface area required for epithelialization.[25,33] They additionally secrete the regulatory enzymes, matrix metalloproteinases, and tissue inhibitors of metalloproteinases, key in the continued remodeling of the extracellular matrix.[31,32] The type III collagen initially deposited by the fibroblasts to form the granulation tissue ultimately is remodeled to type I collagen.[25,30–32] As type I collagen levels increase, the tensile strength of the wound increases up to approximately 80% of preinjury strength by 5 weeks.[25] Although scar remodeling continues for a significantly longer period, the wound site never achieves preinjury strength.[25] During this process, epithelial cells continue to migrate from the periphery, synthesizing a new epithelium and resurfacing the wound.[25] The wound healing process is summarized in **Figs. 4** and **5**.

ACELLULAR DERMAL MATRIX INTEGRATION

A DRT is an inert biomaterial scaffold composed of nonliving dermal components from either allogenic (human cadaver) or xenogenic (animal) origin.[34] The templates serve as the framework to promote the ingrowth of the surrounding host tissues to form a new dermal layer over exposed critical structures.[12,13,34–37] These scaffolds lack an epidermal component and are not used as a skin substitute. They have an outer silicone layer, however, that serves as a barrier to retain moisture and prevent infection, functioning as the epidermis.

The incorporation of the DRT occurs through 4 distinct phases, similar to that of a split-thickness skin graft. These phases consist of imbibition, fibroblast migration, neovascularization, and remodeling/maturation.[38] Imbibition occurs within minutes of application from surrounding wound exudate and quickly leads to graft swelling as it passively absorbs nutrients, cells, and growth factors through diffusion from the surrounding vascularized host tissues.[38] Imbibition from the immediately underlying tissues is not necessary for successful graft incorporation as long as the peripheral tissues have an adequate blood supply to allow for creeping substitution of the graft and creation of a neodermis over avascular structures.[39] Fibroblast migration begins to occur around day 7, leading to further collagen deposition and extracellular matrix creation, with eventual myofibroblast differentiation at approximately day 21.[38] Although myofibroblasts are present, they are in a lesser quantity and without their normal function of wound contraction.[40] During the fourth week, host collagen continues to replace the graft collagen.[38] The fibroblasts remodel the matrix and deposit collagen to create a neodermis.[38] The neodermis then is fully vascularized by the end of week 4 and capable of epithelialization or split-thickness skin graft application.[38] This process of integration is summarized in **Table 2**.

INDICATIONS, CONTRAINDICATIONS, AND APPLICATION

DRTs originally were developed for use in burn injury.[8–11] Since their conception, DRTs indications have been widely expanded for use in a variety of wounds. They effectively recreate a dermal layer that is amendable to skin grafting. The dermal substitute

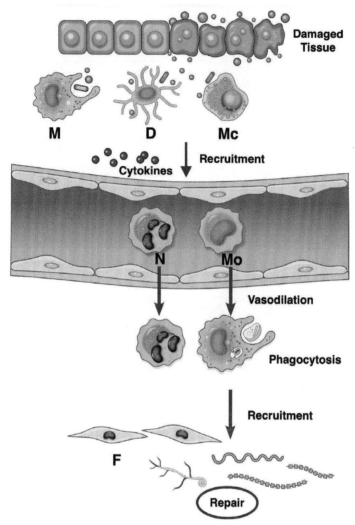

Fig. 4. Aged tissues begin the inflammatory cascade and are recognized by local phagocytic cells, releasing cytokines to further induce progression through the wound healing cascade. The cytokines recruit additional phagocytic cells to the injured site to remove the damaged tissues and further recruit cells capable of producing the building blocks necessary for the repair or regenerative processes, such as fibroblasts (F). D, dendrite; M, macrophage; Mc, monocyte; N, neutrophil. (*Courtesy of* S. Masadeh, DPM, Cincinnati, OH.)

creates an elastic layer that allows for gliding of the skin over muscle flaps or at the donor site of a fasciocutaneous flap.[41,42] Due to this elastic property of the neodermis, DRTs can be applied over joints to reduce contracture.[41,42]

The key components to successful DRT application and incorporation are adequate blood supply to the extremity, complete excision of nonviable or necrotic tissue to create an infection free wound bed as well as uniform wound topography.[43] Appropriate tissue cultures and antibiotic therapy are indicated prior to DRT application.[43] Post-débridement hemostasis is paramount to prevent hematoma formation under

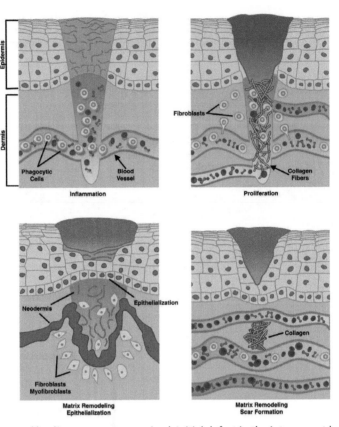

Fig. 5. The wound healing process summarized. Initial defect in the integument leads to the initiation of the cascade with local phagocytic cells and platelets releasing various cytokines to recruit the cells, including fibroblasts and myofibroblasts, involved in the repair process. This results in the formation of a neodermis and eventual epithelialization of the defect. Depending on depth of wound, repair (scar formation) or regeneration may occur. (*Courtesy of* S. Masadeh, DPM, Cincinnati, OH.)

the graft to avoid failure and infection.[44] If the graft is to be applied overlying a joint, the joint should be placed in maximum extension to help reduce contracture.[44] The limb then must be immobilized for a short period of time to prevent motion at the joint and shearing forces across the graft site as incorporation occurs. The graft is secured to the wound with either surgical staples or sutures. The entire application and grafting process is visualized in **Figs. 6–8**. Appropriate surgical dressings also are critical to minimize shear forces, to prevent hematoma or seroma formation, and for promotion of maximum surface area contact. Commonly used postoperative dressings consist of antimicrobial or nonadherent gauze followed by either a bolster, tie-over, or negative-pressure wound device.[44]

If the DRT has an outer silicone layer, it often is removed after suture or staple removal. If the silicone layer does not separate freely, the graft may not have incorporated sufficiently and the silicone layer should be left intact for an additional week. After the removal of the silicone layer, light débridement to the superficial neodermis

Table 2	
Incorporation stages of a dermal regenerative template	
Step 1	The graft and the outer synthetic layer are applied to previously débrided wound site. Synthetic layer prevents environmental exposure and lowers the risk for infection. Graft and silicone layer additionally maintain a moist environment, conducive to healing, and prevent primary contracture, avoiding scar tissue formation.
Step 2	The bodies wound healing cellular mechanisms are activated and invade the template matrix.
Step 3	The graft matrix is replaced by the formation of the neodermis and further deposition of host collagen.
Step 4	The protective outer silicone layer is removed as the newly formed dermis has developed to provide a stable wound construct. The silicone layer is removed easily as the underlying matrix is fully incorporated.
Step 5	The wound site now is suitable for skin grafting or secondary intention healing due to the presence of newly vascularized tissues.

should be performed to prepare the site for split-thickness skin grafting. The silicone layer is maintained until the application of a split-thickness skin graft.

Common complications that may arise after DRT application include hematoma, seroma, infection, and graft shear.[44–46] Hematomas and seromas should be evacuated immediately through either aspiration or perforation of the graft site. Infections need to be treated aggressively with thorough débridement and culture guided antibiosis to avoid graft failure.

DISCUSSION

DRTs have been utilized successfully for soft tissue deficits of the head and neck, chest, pelvis, breast, abdomen, and extremities.[25,42,45–59] In the extremity, grafts have been used as an alternative to flap surgery for wounds where coverage of bone, joint, or tendon is difficult.[1,42,48–53,55,56,59] They recreate a histologic and functional dermis similar to host tissue. This provides improved function and aesthetics to skin grafted wounds.[1,60,61] DRTs provide a framework for native cells to proliferate and decreases the need for myofibroblasts, reducing wound contractures.[40] Shores and colleagues[42] prospectively evaluated 42 patients with exposed tendon void of paratenon in both the upper extremity and lower extremity, with an average wound size of 65 cm^2. Patients had successful wound coverage 92% of the time and retained 91.2% of active range of motion compared with the uninjured contralateral limb.[42] Taras and colleagues[59] additionally evaluated the use of a bilayer dermal matrix for coverage of wounds of the hand with exposed tendon, bone, joint capsule, or hardware and experienced a 95% rate of wound healing utilizing DRTs.

DRTs are versatile in the management of lower extremity wounds in patients with diabetes[43,51,62] Chung and colleagues[51] performed a randomized controlled trial on nonhealing wounds in 307 patients with diabetes evaluating the potential benefit of a bilayer acellular dermal graft. These patients had failed conservative standard of care therapy for 14 days and were appropriately offloaded during the treatment phase. Patients being treated with the graft showed an increased rate of wound closure, improvement in measures in quality of life, and a lower rate of significant adverse events compared with the control group.[51] Faglia and colleagues[62] evaluated the utility of a dermal substitute in diabetic patients who required a partial amputation of the foot. They compared the level of amputation that would be required for primary wound

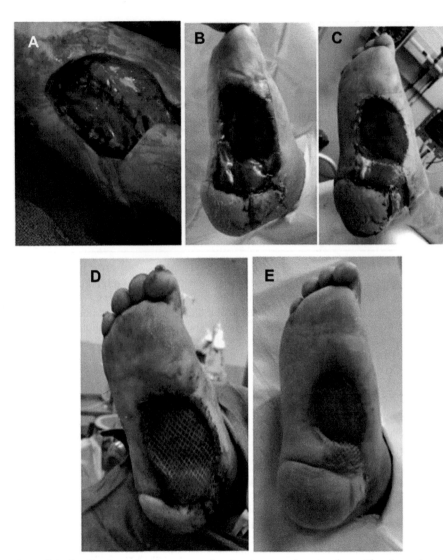

Fig. 6. (*A*) Visualized are the deep avascular structures, such as tendon without paratenon, exposed after initial elevation of the medial plantar artery flap. (*B*) Demonstrates the application of the DRT to the donor site. (*C*) Visualizes the granular tissue and the vascularized wound bed created through the use of the graft after removal of the outer silicone layer. (*D*) Application of split-thickness skin graft to neodermis after temporization of wound bed is achieved. (*E*) Shows the final product with a skin grafted arch and complete healing of both the donor and recipient sites. (*Courtesy of* S. Masadeh, DPM, Cincinnati, OH.)

closure with amputation levels achieved with the use of a DRT.[62] They found a significant decrease in proximal amputation when using these grafts.[62] The preservation of limb length may result in increased function and decreased incidence of recurrent ulceration, lowering the future need for amputation.[62] Marston and colleagues[63] performed a randomized controlled trial evaluating the efficacy of a single-layer dermal regenerative matrix in treating patients with diabetic neuropathic plantar ulcerations.

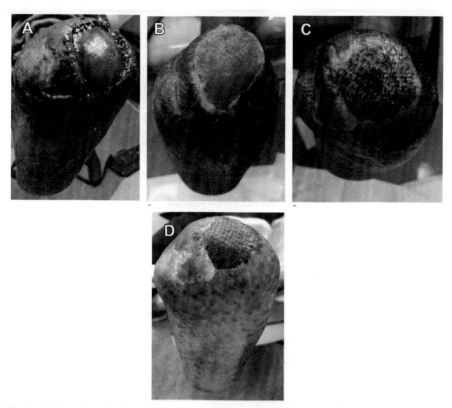

Fig. 7. (*A*) Visualized is the application of a DRT over exposed deep avascular structures after thorough débridement of previous amputation site. (*B*) Shows the granular wound bed that is created after DRT, and wound VAC is utilized. (*C*) demonstrates that acceptance of a split-thickness skin graft from the vascularized wound bed that was created. (*D*) The end result after full healing is achieved. (*Courtesy of* S. Masadeh, DPM, Cincinnati, OH.)

Patients treated with the dermal graft demonstrated a significantly greater proportion and rate of healing compared with the control group.[63] Iorio and colleagues[43] additionally evaluated the use of a bilayer DRT in consecutive patients with diabetes and foot ulcerations requiring surgical intervention to preserve limb length and function. They found that the use of a bilayer template assisted in limb salvage of patients with adequate blood flow and proper infection control.[43] Shakir and colleagues[39] performed a multidisciplinary case-control study evaluating 191 wounds in 147 subjects after the application of a collagen-based DRT for lower extremity reconstruction. They found a statistically significant rate of failure in wounds with either exposed tendon or bone in addition to those wounds present in patients with diabetes and/or surrounding cellulitis.[39] This was supported further in a study performed by Evans and colleagues,[53] in which they found that optimal lower extremity reconstruction occurred in wounds with less than 1 cm of exposed tendon, intact paratenon, and surrounding granulation tissue. This may be attributed to the increased vascularity of the underlying tissues establishing a more accepting wound bed for incorporation.[53] Additionally, Shakir and colleagues[53] found that there was no significant difference in outcomes between the various surgical specialties included in their study, including podiatry, orthopedics, vascular, and plastic surgery.

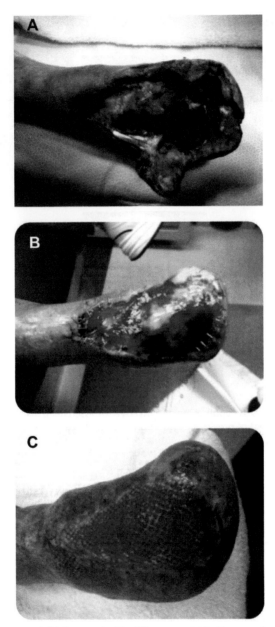

Fig. 8. (*A*) Demonstrates initial wound with diffuse nonviable tissue and exposed deep avascular structures. (*B*) Post-débridement application of bilayer DRT with silicone layer face outwards. (*C*) Represents the endpoint prior to split-thickness skin grafting. (*Courtesy of* S. Masadeh, DPM, Cincinnati, OH.)

SUMMARY

DRT grafts are an evolving group of products that serve as a biodegradable temporizing matrix for the formation of a neodermis. Skin grafting along with local, regional, and free flaps remain valuable tools in managing soft tissue deficits with exposed avascular structures. DRTs have added an intermediary option in treating these wounds, with minimal morbidity to the patient. Current literature is encouraging, although there still is a need for further high-quality trials to truly determine the optimal use of these products. As the indications and efficacies of these products are truly determined, surgeons need to be familiar with their use to optimize patient outcomes and minimize morbidity.

CLINICAL CARE POINTS

- DRTs recreate a dermal layer for the coverage of exposed deep structures, such as bone, tendon, and joint capsule.
- DRTs serve as scaffolds to promote host cell migration, forming a vascularized wound bed.
- DRTs recreate a dermis with similar elastic properties to host tissue, improving mobility and reducing contracture of skin grafts.
- DRTs success is based on appropriate patient selection and excellent wound bed preparation.

DISCLOSURE

The authors have nothing to disclose.

REFERENCES

1. Ellis CV, Kulber DA. Acellular dermal matrices in hand reconstruction. Plast Reconstr Surg 2012;130(5):256–69.
2. Erba P, Ogawa R, Vyas R, et al. The reconstructive matrix: a new paradigm in reconstructive plastic surgery. Plast Reconstr Surg 2010;126:492–8.
3. Gottlieb LJ, Krieger LM. From the reconstructive ladder to the reconstructive elevator. Plast Reconstr Surg 1994;93:1503–4.
4. Mathes SJ, Nahai F. Reconstructive surgery: principles, anatomy & technique, vol. 2. New York: Churchill Livingstone; 1997. Quality Medical.
5. Wong CJ, Niranjan N. Reconstructive stages as an alternative to the reconstructive ladder. Plast Reconstr Surg 2008;121:362–3.
6. Thornton BP, Rosenblum WJ, Lee L. Reconstruction of limited soft-tissue defect with open tibial fracture in the distal third of the leg. Ann Plast Surg 2005;54(3): 276–80.
7. Janis JE, Kwon RK, Attinger CE. The new reconstructive ladder: modifications to the traditional model. Plast Reconstr Surg 2011;127:205–12.
8. Heimbach D, Luterman A, Burke J, et al. Artificial dermis for major burns: a multicenter randomized clinical trial. Ann Surg 1988;208:313–20.
9. Yannas IV, Burke JF. Design of an artificial skin. I. Basic design principles. J Biomed Mater Res 1980;14(01):65–81.
10. Yannas IV, Burke JF, Gordon PL, et al. Design of an artificial skin. II. Control of chemical composition. J Biomed Mater Res 1980;14(02):107–32.
11. Dagalakis N, Flink J, Stasikelis P, et al. Design of an artificial skin: III. Control of pore structure. J Biomed Mater Res 1980;14:511.

12. Banyard DA, Bourgeois JM, Widgerow AD, et al. Regenerative biomaterials: a review. Plast Reconstr Surg 2015;135(06):1740–8.
13. Tenenhaus M, Rennekampff HO. Current concepts in tissue engineering: skin and wound. Plast Reconstr Surg 2016;138(3):42–50.
14. Myers S, Navaria H, Ojeh N. Skin Engineering and Keratinocyte Stem Cell Therapy. Tissue Engineering (2nd Edition). 2014: 497-528.
15. Benson HAE, Watkinson AC. (2012). Transdermal and Topical Drug Delivery: Principles and Practice.
16. Doughty DB, McNichol LL. (2015). Wound, Ostomy and Continence Nurses society core curriculum: Wound management.
17. Feldman R, Maibach HI. Absorption of some organic compounds through the skin in man. J Invest Dermatol 1970;54:399–404.
18. Lee SH, Jeong SK, Ahn SK. An update of the defensive barrier function of skin. Yonsei Med J 2006;47(3):293–306.
19. Brodell LA, Rosenthal KS. Skin structure and function the body's primary defense against infection. Infect Dis Clin Pract 2008;16:113–7.
20. Bruckner-Tuderman L, Hopfner B, Hammami-Hauasli N. Biology of anchoring fibrils: lessons from dystrophic epidermolysis bullosa. Matrix Biol 1999;18(1): 43–54.
21. Halata Z, Grim M, Bauman KI. Friedrich Sigmund Merkel and his "Merkel cell" morphology, development, and physiology: review and new results. Anat Rec A Discov Mol Cell Evol Biol 2003;271(1):225–39.
22. Eming SA, Martin P, Tomic Canic M. Wound repair and regeneration: mechanisms, signaling, and translation. Sci Transl Med 2014;6(265):1–36.
23. Kumar V, Abbas AK, Aster JC, et al. Robbins basic pathology. Philadelphia: Elsevier/Saunders; 2013. Chapters 2 and 3.
24. Broughton G, Janis JE, Attinger CE. The basic science of wound healing. Plast Reconstr Surg 2006;117(7):12–34.
25. Janis JE, Harrison B. Wound healing: part I. Basic science. Plast Reconstr Surg 2016;138(3):9–17.
26. Mohd J, Effat Omar YS, Pai DR, et al. Cellular events and Biomarkers of wound healing. Indian J Plast Surg 2012;45(2):220–8.
27. Singer AJ, Clark RA. Cutaneous wound healing. N Engl J Med 1999;341:738–46.
28. Ganapathy N, Subramaniyan Venkataraman S, Daniel R, et al. Molecular biology of wound healing. J Pharm Bioallied Sci 2012;4(2):334–7.
29. Albelda SM, Buck CA. Integrins and other cell adhesion molecules. FASEB J 1990;4:2868–80.
30. Clark RAF, Nielsen LD, Welch MP, et al. Collagen matrices attenuate the collagen-synthetic response of cultured fibroblasts to TGF-b. J Cell Sci 1995;108:1251–61.
31. Bochaton-Piallat ML, Gabbiani G, Hinz B. The myofibroblast in wound healing and fibrosis: answered and unanswered questions. F1000 Res 2016;5:1–8.
32. Darby I, Laverdet B, Bonte F, et al. Fibroblasts and myofibroblasts in wound healing. Clin Cosmet Investig Dermatol 2014;7:301–11.
33. Berry DP, Harding KG, Stanton MR, et al. Human wound contraction: collagen organization, fibroblasts, and myofibroblasts. Plast Reconstr Surg 1998;102(1): 124–31.
34. Tork S, Jefferson R, Janis J. Acellular dermal matrices: applications in plastic surgery. Semin Plast Surg 2019;33:173–84.
35. Badylak SF. The extracellular matrix as a scaffold for tissue reconstruction. Semin Cell Dev Biol 2002;13(05):377–83.

36. Wan D, Potter JK. Biomaterials. In: Janis JE, editor. Essentials of plastic surgery. 2nd edition. Boca Raton (FL): CRC Press; 2016. p. 87–104.
37. Novitsky YW, Rosen MJ. The biology of biologics: basic science and clinical concepts. Plast Reconstr Surg 2012;130(05):9–17.
38. Moiemen NS, Vlachou E, Staiano JJ, et al. Reconstructive surgery with Integra dermal regeneration template: histologic study, clinical evaluation, and current practice. Plast Reconstr Surg 2006;117(7):160–74.
39. Shakir S, Messa CA, Broach RB, et al. Indications and limitations of bilayer wound matrix-based lower extremity reconstruction: a multidisciplinary case-control study of 191 wounds. Plast Reconstr Surg 2020;145(3):813–22.
40. Mirastschijski U, Schnabel R, Claes J, et al. Matrix metalloproteinase inhibition delays wound healing and blocks the latent transforming growth factor-b1-promoted myofibroblast formation and function. Wound Repair Regen 2010;18: 223–34.
41. Kim YJ, Kim MY, Lee PK, et al. Evaluation of natural change of skin function in split-thickness skin grafts by noninvasive bioengineering methods. Dermatol Surg 2006;32:1358–63.
42. Shores JT, Hiersche M, Gabriel A, et al. Tendon coverage using an artificial skin substitute. J Plast Reconstr Aesthet Surg 2012;65:1544–50.
43. Iorio ML, Goldstein J, Adams M, et al. Functional limb salvage in the diabetic patient: the use of a collagen bilayer matrix and risk factors for amputation. Plast Reconstr Surg 2011;127:260–7.
44. Change DK, Louis MR, Gimenez A, et al. The basics of integra dermal regeneration template and its expanding clinical applications. Semin Plast Surg 2019; 33(3):185–9.
45. Chalmers RL, Smock E, Geh JLC. Experience of Integra in cancer reconstructive surgery. J Plast Reconstr Aesthet Surg 2010;63(12):2081–90.
46. Dantzer E, Braye FM. Reconstructive surgery using an artificial dermis (Integra): results with 39 grafts. Br J Plast Surg 2001;54(08):659–64.
47. Abai B, Thayer D, Glat PM. The use of a dermal regeneration template (Integra) for acute resurfacing and reconstruction of defects created by excision of giant hairy nevi. Plast Reconstr Surg 2004;114(01):162–8.
48. Barcot Z, Dakovic Bacalja I, Zupancic B, et al. Treating giant congenital nevus with integra dermal regeneration template in a 9-year-old girl. Int J Low Extrem Wounds 2017;16(02):143–5.
49. Bidic SM, Dauwe PB, Heller J, et al. Reconstructing large keloids with neodermis: a systematic review. Plast Reconstr Surg 2012;129(02):380e–2e.
50. Clayman MA, Clayman SM, Mozingo DW. The use of collagen-glycosaminoglycan copolymer (Integra) for the repair of hypertrophic scars and keloids. J Burn Care Res 2006;27(03):404–9.
51. Driver VR, Lavery LA, Reyzelman AM, et al. A clinical trial of Integra Template for diabetic foot ulcer treatment. Wound Repair Regen 2015;23(06):891–900.
52. Frame JD, Still J, Lakhel-LeCoadou A, et al. Use of dermal regeneration template in contracture release procedures: a multicenter evaluation. Plast Reconstr Surg 2004;113(05):1330–8.
53. Kim PJ, Attinger CE, Steinberg JS, et al. Integra bilayer wound matrix application for complex lower extremity soft tissue reconstruction. Surg Technol Int 2014;24: 65–73.
54. Komorowska-Timek E, Gabriel A, Bennett DC, et al. Artificial dermis as an alternative for coverage of complex scalp defects following excision of malignant tumors. Plast Reconstr Surg 2005;115(04):1010–7.

55. Reynolds M, Kelly DA, Walker NJ, et al. Use of Integra in the management of complex hand wounds from cancer resection and nonburn trauma. Hand (N Y) 2018; 13(01):74–9.

56. Senchenkov A. Reconstruction of radial forearm donor-site defects with Integra and staged full-thickness skin graft. Plast Reconstr Surg 2013;132(05):884–6.

57. Stiefel D, Schiestl C, Meuli M. Integra Artificial Skin for burn scar revision in adolescents and children. Burns 2010;36(01):114–20.

58. Su JJ, Chang DK, Mailey B, et al. Treatment of a giant congenital melanocytic nevus in the adult: review of the current management of giant congenital melanocytic nevus. Ann Plast Surg 2015;74(Suppl. 01):57–61.

59. Taras JS, Sapienza A, Roach JB, et al. Acellular dermal regeneration template for soft tissue reconstruction of the digits. J Hand Surg Am 2010;35(03):415–21.

60. Sinha UK, Shih C, Chang K, et al. Use of AlloDerm for coverage of radial forearm free flap donor site. Laryngoscope 2002;112(02):230–4.

61. Wax MK, Winslow CP, Andersen PE. Use of allogenic dermis for radial forearm free flap donor site coverage. J Otolaryngol 2002;31(06):341–5.

62. Clerici G, Caminiti M, Curci V, et al. The use of a dermal substitute to preserve maximal foot length in diabetic foot wounds with tendon and bone exposure following urgent surgical debridement for acute infection. Int J Wound 2020; 7(3):176–83.

63. Frykberg RG, Marston WA, Cardinal M. The incidence of lower-extremity amputation and bone resection in diabetic foot ulcer patients treated with a human fibroblast-derived dermal substitute. Adv Skin Wound Care 2015;28(1):17–20.

Skin Graft Techniques

Arshad A. Khan, DPM[a,b,]*, Isra M. Khan, MD[c,d], Phi P. Nguyen, MD[e,f,g],
Erwin Lo, MD[h,i], Hassan Chahadeh, MD[j], Mathew Cerniglia, DPM[k],
James A. Noriega, DPM, CWSP[l]

KEYWORDS

- Wound healing • Orthoplastic • Skin graft • Ulcer • Skin transplantation
- Lower extremity • Split-thickness skin graft

KEY POINTS

- The authors provide a review of literature regarding skin grafting for the treatment of lower extremity traumatic and non-traumatic wounds.
- Harvesting sites are discussed for lower extremity wounds.
- A stepwise approach from harvesting of the graft to its transplantation are reviewed.

INTRODUCTION

The treatment of complex wounds of the lower extremities can be extremely challenging for the lower extremity surgeon. When performing a salvage of the lower extremity it is essential to take into consideration several factors including, osseous defects, infection, neural and vascular status, and soft tissue coverage.[1,2] Implementation of an orthoplastic approach to lower extremity reconstruction has increasingly become an important modality in the management of lower limb defects. There are several approaches and algorithms described in the literature regarding lower extremity salvage techniques. Rodriguez-Collazo and Khan have described an orthoplastic algorithmic approach to wounds associated with distal one-third of the lower extremity.[3–5]

[a] Department of Orthopedic Surgery, Indiana University School of Medicine, Gary/Northwest, Gary, IN, USA; [b] SpineTech Neurosurgeons, SpineTech Brain and Spine of South East Texas, Shenandoah, TX, USA; [c] Chicago Foot and Ankle Deformity Correction Center, Chicago, IL, USA; [d] 111 Vision Park Boulevard, Suite 200, Shenandoah, TX 77384, USA; [e] McGowan Medical School, Houston, TX, USA; [f] MIA Plastic Surgery, 4126 Southwest Fwy Suite 999, Houston, TX 77027, USA; [g] MILA Med Spa Group, Houston, TX, USA; [h] University of Texas Medical Branch, Mischer Neuroscience Institute, Houston, TX, USA; [i] Brain and Spine Center of Southeast Texas, 6025 Metropolitan Drive, Suite 205, Beaumont, TX 77706, USA; [j] Vision Park of Surgery Center, 111 Vision Park Boulevard, Suite 200, Shenandoah, TX 77384, USA; [k] Private Practice, 816 Towne Ct Suite 100, Saginaw, TX 76179, USA; [l] Department of Surgery, LSU School of Medicine, Our Lady of Lourdes Hospital, 203 West Brentwood Boulevard, Suite 2, Lafayette, LA 70506, USA
* Corresponding author. 111 Vision Park Boulevard, Suite 200, Shenandoah, TX 77384.
E-mail address: akhan@spinetech.com

Clin Podiatr Med Surg 37 (2020) 821–835
https://doi.org/10.1016/j.cpm.2020.07.007
0891-8422/20/© 2020 Elsevier Inc. All rights reserved.

There are a variety of lower extremity reconstructive options available for coverage of skin and soft tissue defects such as, flaps and skin grafts. Flaps are a reliable method for coverage of lower limb defects that can be single staged or multiple stages. Cierny and colleagues found that single staged procedures performed on open tibial fractures had a better result than delayed techniques.[6] When primary wound closure is unable to be attained then one must consider the use of skin grafts. In such cases, a split-thickness skin graft (STSG) is often times used as the method of reconstruction. The current standard of care for closure of nonhealing wounds is the use of split thickness skin grafting.[7] This article will focus on the surgical techniques in lower extremity reconstruction with the application of split-thickness skin grafts.

HISTORY

Grafting of skin has been performed for several centuries throughout the world. The Hindu Tilemaker Caste described techniques of skin harvesting and transplantation used for amputated noses after judicial punishment nearly 3000 years ago.[8] G.Baronio in 1804 carried out the transferring of various thickness skin grafts to sheep tails.[9] Sir Astley Paston Cooper, 1st Baronet was an English surgeon and anatomist who performed a procedure by taking the skin from an amputated thumb and using it as coverage for a stump defect in 1817. Reverdin and Thiersch both performed skin grafts on wounds by using pinch grafts in the mid to late 19th century.[7,10] Use of split-thickness grafts were described in the late 19th century by Ollier and Thiersch.[11] Full-thickness grafting was described by Wolfe in 1875 and Krause in 1893 respectively.[9] In their textbook from 1929, Blair and Brown were the first to describe the use of an "intermediate split-thickness graft."[12] In 1946 Padgett described the technique of "thick skin grafting" of patients that had burns. He and his engineering partner, George Hood, created the first mechanical dermatome that was able to create sheets of graft that were 4cm X 8cm.[13] Today skin grafting is used widely in fields of dermatology and plastic surgery.[14–18]

SKIN SUBSTITUTES

Engineering of skin substitutes has been carried out to help cover large defects such as burns. These include acellular biomaterials as well as composite culture skin analogs that contain both allogenic as well as autologous cultured cells. The main characteristics associated with these skin substitutes include wound coverage, prevention of wound infection, and to restore functions and qualities associated with skin. There are currently no skin substitutes that are able to replace all of the functions of intact human skin. A disadvantage of using skin allograft is their high costs and this has led to increased use of xenografts and other types of skin substitutes.[19,20]

ANATOMY

The largest organ of the human body is the skin and accounts for approximately 7% of the body weight of an average individual. The skin has many functions, with its main roles being to serve as a protective barrier and thermoregulator.[21,22] The skin also has metabolic functions in protein and vitamin D metabolism. Approximately 95% of the skin is made up of the dermis with the remaining 5% being the epidermis. The epidermis is the thin external outer layer which is composed of mainly stratified squamous epithelium and keratinocytes. The dermis is the thick inner layer composed of connective tissue, collagen, sweat glands, hair follicles and a layer of subcutaneous fat called the hypodermis.[22]

The nature of skin varies with each individual depending on age, amount of sun exposure and the particular location of skin.[22] Skin grafting requires a reliable vascular supply to ensure tissue survival and a good donor match for an adequate aesthetic result.[23,24] Cutaneous vasculature comes from the dermis and hypodermis, while the epidermis is an avascular tissue. Cutaneous vessels arise from branches of the underlying muscle vessels which penetrate the subcutaneous fat ascending to the dermis and epidermis respectively.[22]

Properties of Skin Grafts

Generally grafts can be divided into 4 categories: autografts, allografts, xenografts, and artificial skin or bioengineered skin.

- Autografts
  - Skin that is directly taken from the patient
- Allografts
  - Skin that is from a human donor
- Xenografts
  - Skin taken from an animal
- Bioengineered
  - This is skin that is engineered and cultured in a lab

The success skin grafting corresponds to the blood supply of the skin from which the graft was harvested and the metabolic activity of the skin graft at the time of its application. Grafts obtained from highly vascularized donor sites typically heal better than those of a poorly perfused area. Metabolic activity of the skin graft at the time of application correlates to the tolerance the graft will have during the period of ischemia.[24,25]

Graft take is the process by which the graft is incorporated in the host bed.[22] The three phases of skin graft take include plasmatic inhibition, inosculatory phase, and a capillary growth phase. Plasmatic inhibition is the first phase, lasting a period of 24-48 hours. Following this, the inosculatory phase and capillary growth take place concurrently until the fifth or sixth post-graft day when generalized blood flow has been established.[22,26]

PROPERTIES OF SKIN AUTOGRAFTS

Full-thickness Skin Grafts
- Composed of entire dermis as well as the epidermis
- Typically indicated for small areas
- Minimal risk of contracture

Split-thickness Skin Grafts
- Composed of the entire epidermis and a superficial portion of the dermis
- Typically indicated for large areas; areas too large for use of a flap or FTSG
- Three thickness types may be used depending on the amount of dermis taken
  - Thin: .008-.012 inches
  - Medium/Intermediate: .013-.016 inches
  - Thick: .017-.02 inches
- Increased risk of contracture and painful donor sites in comparison to FTSG.[23,24,27]

Split-thickness skin grafts serve as protection to the host bed from further trauma while also providing a barrier to infection. To prevent infection, STSG require placement on well-vascularized beds with a low bacterial count.[22,26] Wound closure with

STSG is a versatile method of skin grafting due to its ability to survive on relatively avascular sites. Donor sites for STSG are large and typically harvested from the outer thigh due to its technical ease and convenience of positioning intraoperatively and postoperatively for dressings.[24]

PREOPERATIVE PLANNING

Prior to surgical intervention it is important to identify any underlying causes that may affect graft adherence to the recipient bed. This include the patients co morbidities and possible infection. Contraindications to skin grafting include poor blood supply to the wound bed, insufficient soft tissue coverage with exposed tendon, exposed bone or exposed nerve.[28]

Once these have been addressed then the surgeon may move forward and determine donor site location. It is important to first identify which type of skin graft will be utilized, meshed, sheet (unmeshed), pinch type or lab cultured skin grafts. Each of these types of grafts requires a different type of harvesting method and may require specific instrumentation. This paper will be specifically discussing skin graft techniques in regards to harvesting and transplantation of the split-thickness autograft to a recipient wound bed of the lower extremity.

DONOR SITE PREPARATION

Donor site is determined after measuring the wound site and taking in to account the length, width, and depth of the recipient wound site. This will allow the surgeon to identify the amount of skin graft needed. Other considerations for identifying a donor site include skin thickness, pigmentation, ease of harvest, patient position and aesthetics

Donor sites can include back, buttocks, inguinal ligament region, anterolateral thigh, outer thigh, the popliteal fossa, the posterior calf, the lateral malleolus, dorsal foot and plantar medial arch of the foot. The authors preference for lower extremity coverage is from the lateral thigh or posterior calf.[29]

TRANSPLANTATION SITE PREPARATION

The recipient bed must be prepared by removal of all non-viable tissues and undermining as needed. This can be accomplished by meticulous debridement using biological, hydro-surgical and or chemical techniques. Hemostasis should be performed of all venous bleeders. The wound bed preparation can be single staged or a delayed method. Once good vascularity and clean wound margins are identified one can proceed with transplantation of skin graft to the recipient bed.[30,31]

PROCEDURAL APPROACH

Instrumentation/Equipment/Materials:
- Lidocaine with epinephrine
- Sterile mineral oil or sterile saline
- Dermatome or Humby knife
- Tissue forceps
- Scissor
- Graft Mesher
- Sterile saline
- Soft guaze
- Vasiline guaze

- Skin staples
- Suture

HARVESTING TECHNIQUE/TRANSPLANTATION TECHNIQUE
Step 1

The patient brought into the operating room and placed on the operating room table in the supine position. Attention is then directed to the harvest site which is prepped and draped in the usual sterile manner.

Step 2

Using a marking pen and the measurements obtained from the wound bed the dimensions are drawn out at the graft harvest site and a dermatome template is selected (**Fig. 1**). The graft size is now selected on the dermatome and the authors preferred size is 0.018 of an inch for lower extremity split-thickness skin grafting (**Fig. 2**).

Step 3

Anesthesia is obtained at the harvest site by injecting 1% lidocaine with epinephrine mixed with 10 cc of saline to help increase the turgor. This mixture helps to create anesthesia, hemostasis and also helps with trans-sectioning of the hair follicles (**Fig. 3**).

Step 4

Sterile mineral oil is also used to prep the harvest site and used for lining the blade and template on the dermatome.

Step 5

Tension is now created at the donor site by using either tongue depressors at the proximal and distal edges of the graft harvesting site or by using 4 towel clamps to create tension at the 4 edges of the donor site (**Figs. 4** and **5**).

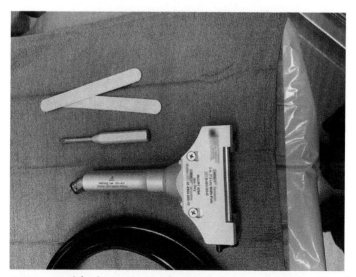

Fig. 1. Dermatome used for harvesting graft and sterile tongue depressors used to create tension at the harvesting site.

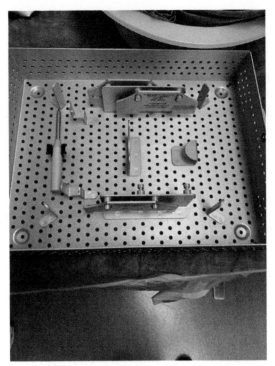

Fig. 2. Templates used for identifying the correct size for graft harvesting.

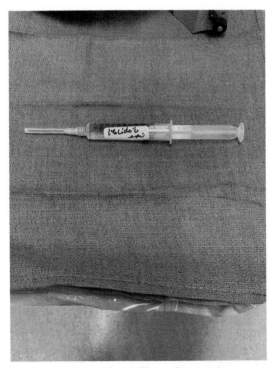

Fig. 3. Lidocaine with epinephrine used to infiltrate harvest site.

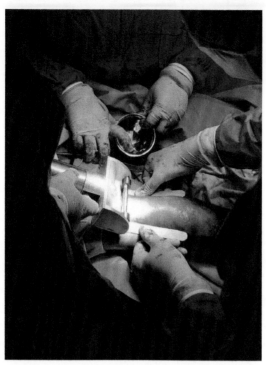

Fig. 4. Tongue depressors are used to create tension when using dermatome to harvest graft.

Step 6

A mechanical dermatome is used at the proximal aspect of the graft site at an approximately a 45 degree angle and slowly progressed forward toward the skin edge. Once the blade engages the skin you will decrease the angle and continue to move toward the distal graft border in an almost parallel fashion. Once the distal edge is reached the dermatome is now directed upward slowly and the skin is released from the site. Graft harvesting should be performed using one consecutive motion throughout the procedure. It is also important to have an assistant hold the harvested skin as it comes through the dermatome to prevent it from getting caught back into the blade. This can be accomplished by using two Adson tissue forceps and care must be taken to prevent tearing of the harvested skin.

Step 7

Once the skin graft has been obtained it is now placed now on a skin graft carrier with the dermal side up. You will need to use some saline to help unravel graft edges as it is place on carrier. It is important to use a marking pen to mark the dermal side of the graft to prevent placing the graft in an improper orientation with the epidermal side down at the recipient site.

Step 8

The skin graft with the carrier is now placed through the mesher using a 1.5:1 mesh (**Fig. 6**). It is important to tease away the graft from the mesher to prevent shredding.

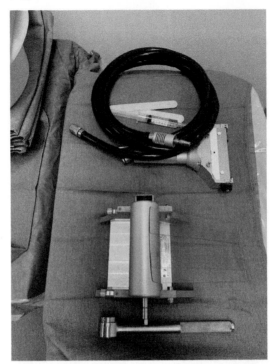

Fig. 5. Items used when harvesting a split-thickness skin graft include a dermatome, 2 sterile tongue depressors, Lidocaine with epinephrine, a mesher and mineral oil not shown here.

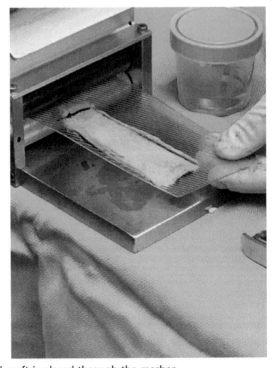

Fig. 6. Harvested graft is placed through the mesher.

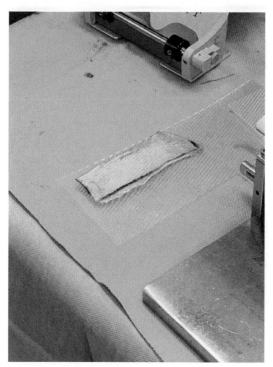

Fig. 7. Harvested graft is placed on mesher tray with the dermal side facing up.

Once this is complete a saline soaked gauze is placed over the graft on top of the carrier with the dermal side now up on the gauze (**Fig. 7**). If there is no mesher available one can use a #11 blade and use a "pie crusted" method to create fenestrations in the graft.

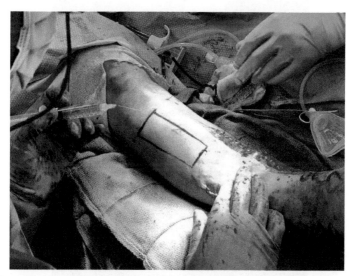

Fig. 8. Measurement and marking of a Split thickness skin graft harvested from the lateral lower leg.

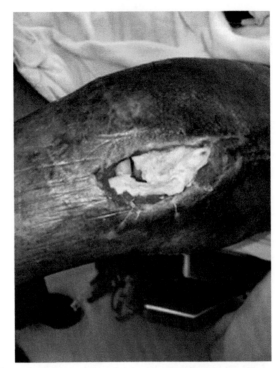

Fig. 9. Exposed knee replacement that has not healed for greater than a year.

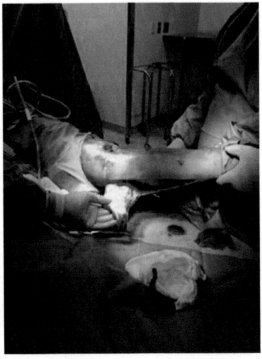

Fig. 10. Harvested gastroc muscle for coverage of exposed knee wound and replacement.

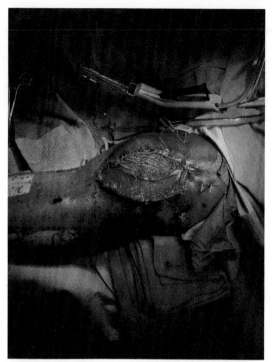

Fig. 11. Transplantation of harvested Split-thickness graft after gastroc muscle flap for exposed knee replacement.

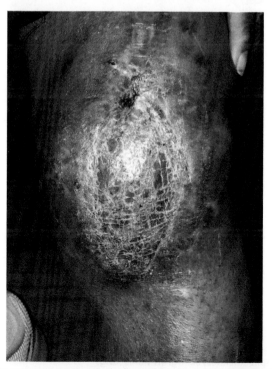

Fig. 12. Six months postop gastroc muscle flap with split-thickness graft transplantation.

Step 9

The graft is now positioned next to the recipient site which should have already been prepared and cleansed, and placed directly on to the wound bed. Care is once again taken to identify the dermis which is placed toward the wound (**Fig. 8**). There are multiple forms of fixation that can be applied to hold the skin graft in place, these include sutures, staples, and steri-strips.

Step 10

Once the graft has been transplanted to the recipient bed a stent type dressing is applied to help the skin graft to adhere directly to the wound bed providing continuous pressure and helping to prevent hematoma and sheer forces. Post operative Dressings are applied consisting of sterile gauze, an ABD pad, and soft dressing roll.

RECOVERY AND MANAGEMENT

It is important to continue to care for both the donor site as well as the transplantation site. The authors usually leave the dressings intact and change them at approximately

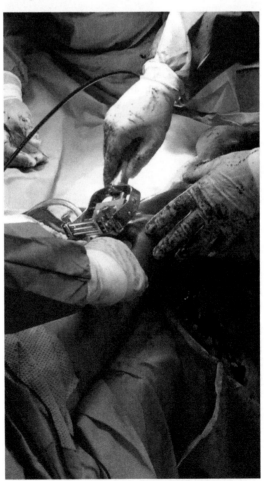

Fig. 13. Video of split-thickness skin graft harvesting.

5-7 days post-op. Patient should be notified that they may experience increased pain at the donor site initially after their procedure. Serebarkian, and colleagues found in their meta-analysis, by using moist dressings a reduction in pain was identified as well as better re-epithelialization rates.[32]

COMPLICATIONS

Possible complications associated with split-thickness skin grafting include loss of grafted skin due to excessive bleeding causing hematoma, excessive motion with sheer forces and infection at the transposition site (**Fig. 9**). Other complications can occur such as skin discoloration, scar tissue formation, loss of sensation, venous thrombosis and uneven surface.[33] Infections associated with skin graft loss are more commonly found with vascular ulcers, burns, lower extremity application and when grafting is performed at multiple sites. Pseudomonas aeruginosa was the most commonly cultured microbe found with infected skin grafts followed by Staphylococcus aureus. Teh found that specific bacteria at the graft site produced proteolytic enzymes that resulted in the failure of the skin graft. Full thickness skin grafts were noted to be less susceptible to infection when compared to split-thickness skin grafts (**Figs. 10–13**).[34,35]

SUMMARY

Skin grafting is an important adjunct for lower extremity wounds related to trauma and ulcerations. Skin grafting is an important tool that surgeons who perform complex lower extremity limb salvage and wound management should have in their skill set. The surgeon should become comfortable with the techniques outlined in this paper in regards to skin graft harvesting of split-thickness skin grafts as well their transplantation to the recipient wound bed. It is also important to identify and stabilize all comorbidities prior to performing these procedures in order to help limit complications associated with skin grafting. Pre-operative planning as well as post-operative management in regards to the harvest site and recipient bed management are crucial for successful skin grafting. Skin grafting is a reliable procedure for providing coverage for deficits associated with lower extremity wounds.

DISCLOSURE

No funding was received for this publication and there are no conflicts of interest.

REFERENCES

1. Kadam D. Limb salvage surgery. Indian J Plast Surg 2013;46(2):265–74.
2. Mendenhall SD, Ben-Amotz O, Gandhi RA, et al. A review on the orthoplastic approach to lower limb reconstruction. Indian J Plast Surg 2019;52(1):17–25.
3. Rodriguez-Collazo E, Khan AA, Khan HA. An algorithmic approach towards the orthoplastic management of osseous and soft tissue defects in post-traumatic distal tibial fractures. J Orthop Trauma Surg Relat Res 2017;12(2):57–61.
4. Azoury SC, Stranix JT, Kovach SJ, et al. Principles of orthoplastic surgery for lower extremity reconstruction: why is this important? J Reconstr Microsurg 2019. https://doi.org/10.1055/s-0039-1695753.
5. Langer V. Management of major limb injuries. ScientificWorldJournal 2014;2014: 640430.

6. Cierny G 3rd, Byrd HS, Jones RE. Primary versus delayed soft tissue coverage for severe open tibial fractures. A comparison of results. Clin Orthop Relat Res 1983;(178):54–63.

7. Thorne C, Gurtner G, Chung K, et al. Grabb and Smith's plastic surgery. Philadelphia: Wolters Kluwer Health/Lippincott Williams & Wilkins; 2013.

8. Hauben DJ, Baruchin A, Mahler A. On the history of the free skin graft. Ann Plast Surg 1982;9(3):242–5.

9. Davis JS. The story of plastic surgery. Ann Surg 1994;113:641.

10. Tiersch C. Über Hautverplanzung. Verh Dtsch Ges Chir 1886;15-17.

11. Davis JS. Address of the president: the story of plastic surgery. Ann Surg 1941; 113(5):641–56.

12. Smahel J. The healing of skin grafts. Clin Plast Surg 1977;4(3):409–24.

13. Bennett JE, Miller SR. Evolution of the electro-dermatome. Plast Reconstr Surg 1970;45(2):131–4.

14. Pollack SV. Wound healing: a review. IV. Systemic medications affecting wound healing. J Dermatol Surg Oncol 1982;8(8):667–72.

15. Blair VP, Brown JB. Use and uses of large split skin grafts of intermediate thickness. Surg Gynecol Obstet 1929;49:82–97.

16. Padgett EC. Skin grafting of the burned patient. Plast Reconstr Surg 1946;2(4): 368–74.

17. Shimizu R, Kishi K. Skin graft. Plast Surg Int 2012;2012:563493.

18. Bonifant H, Holloway S. A review of the effects of ageing on skin integrity and wound healing. Br J Community Nurs 2019;24(Sup3):S28–33.

19. Supp DM, Boyce ST. Engineered skin substitutes: practices and potentials. Clin Dermatol 2005;23(4):403–12.

20. Haddad AG, Giatsidis G, Orgill DP, et al. Skin substitutes and bioscaffolds: temporary and permanent coverage. Clin Plast Surg 2017;44(3):627–34.

21. Mccartan B, Dinh T. The use of split-thickness skin grafts on diabetic foot ulcerations: a literature review. Plast Surg Int 2012;2012:1–6.

22. Thornton JF, Gosman AA. Skin grafts and skin substitutes and principles of flaps. Selected Readings Plast Surg 2004;10(1). Available at: srps.org/product/volume-10-issue-1/srps.org/product/volume-10-issue-1/.

23. Choi J-Y, Kim SH, Oh GJ, et al. Management of defects on lower extremities with the use of matriderm and skin graft. Arch Plast Surg 2014;41(4):337. https://doi.org/10.5999/aps.2014.41.4.337.

24. Prohaska J, Cook C. Skin grafting. In: StatPearls. U.S. National Library of Medicine; 2019.

25. Santema TB, Poyck PP, Ubbink DT. Skin grafting and tissue replacement for treating foot ulcers in people with diabetes. Cochrane Database Syst Rev 2016;(2):CD011255.

26. Simman R, Phavixay L. Split-thickness skin grafts remain the gold standard for the closure of large acute and chronic wounds. J Am Col Certif Wound Spec 2011;3(3):55–9.

27. Kanapathy M, Hachach-Haram N, Bystrzonowski N, et al. Epidermal grafting versus split-thickness skin grafting for wound healing (EPIGRAAFT): study protocol for a randomised controlled trial. Trials 2016;17:1. https://doi.org/10.1186/s13063-016-1352-y.

28. Schubert HM, Brandstetter M, Ensat F, et al. Spalthauttransplantation zur weichteildefektdeckung [Split thickness skin graft for coverage of soft tissue defects]. Oper Orthop Traumatol 2012;24(4–5):432–8. https://doi.org/10.1007/s00064-011-0134-7.

29. Coban Y, Aytekin A, Goktekin T. Skin graft harvesting and donor site selection. 2011. https://doi.org/10.5772/21957.
30. Meaume S. Methods of non surgical debridement of wounds in 2011. Soins 2011; 752:44–7.
31. Gabriel A, Wong W, Gupta S. Single-stage reconstruction for soft tissue defects: a case series. Ostomy Wound Manage 2012;58(6):30–7.
32. Serebrakian AT, Pickrell BB, Varon DE, et al. Meta-analysis and systematic review of skin graft donor-site dressings with future guidelines. Plast Reconstr Surg Glob Open 2018;6(9):e1928.
33. Struk S, Correia N, Guenane Y, et al. Full-thickness skin grafts for lower leg defects coverage: interest of postoperative immobilization. Ann Chir Plast Esthet 2018;63(3):229–33.
34. Unal S, Ersoz G, Demirkan F, et al. Analysis of skin-graft loss due to infection: infection-related graft loss. Ann Plast Surg 2005;55(1):102–6.
35. Teh BT. Why do skin grafts fail? Plast Reconstr Surg 1979;63(3):323–32.

UNITED STATES POSTAL SERVICE ®
Statement of Ownership, Management, and Circulation
(All Periodicals Publications Except Requester Publications)

1. Publication Title	2. Publication Number	3. Filing Date
CLINICS IN PODIATRIC MEDICINE & SURGERY	000 – 707	9/18/2020

4. Issue Frequency	5. Number of Issues Published Annually	6. Annual Subscription Price
JAN, APR, JUL, OCT	4	$304.00

7. Complete Mailing Address of Known Office of Publication (Not printer) (Street, city, county, state, and ZIP+4®)

ELSEVIER INC.
230 Park Avenue, Suite 800
New York, NY 10169

Contact Person
Malathi Samayan

Telephone (Include area code)
91-44-4299-4507

8. Complete Mailing Address of Headquarters or General Business Office of Publisher (Not printer)

ELSEVIER INC.
230 Park Avenue, Suite 800
New York, NY 10169

9. Full Names and Complete Mailing Addresses of Publisher, Editor, and Managing Editor (Do not leave blank)

Publisher (Name and complete mailing address)

DOLORES MELONI, ELSEVIER INC.
1600 JOHN F KENNEDY BLVD. SUITE 1800
PHILADELPHIA, PA 19103-2899

Editor (Name and complete mailing address)

LAUREN BOYLE, ELSEVIER INC.
1600 JOHN F KENNEDY BLVD. SUITE 1800
PHILADELPHIA, PA 19103-2899

Managing Editor (Name and complete mailing address)

PATRICK MANLEY, ELSEVIER INC.
1600 JOHN F KENNEDY BLVD. SUITE 1800
PHILADELPHIA, PA 19103-2899

10. Owner (Do not leave blank. If the publication is owned by a corporation, give the name and address of the corporation immediately followed by the names and addresses of all stockholders owning or holding 1 percent or more of the total amount of stock. If not owned by a corporation, give the names and addresses of the individual owners. If owned by a partnership or other unincorporated firm, give its name and address as well as those of each individual owner. If the publication is published by a nonprofit organization, give its name and address.)

Full Name	Complete Mailing Address
WHOLLY OWNED SUBSIDIARY OF REED/ELSEVIER, US HOLDINGS	1600 JOHN F KENNEDY BLVD. SUITE 1800 PHILADELPHIA, PA 19103-2899

11. Known Bondholders, Mortgagees, and Other Security Holders Owning or Holding 1 Percent or More of Total Amount of Bonds, Mortgages, or Other Securities. If none, check box ▶ ☐ None

Full Name	Complete Mailing Address
N/A	

12. Tax Status (For completion by nonprofit organizations authorized to mail at nonprofit rates) (Check one)
The purpose, function, and nonprofit status of this organization and the exempt status for federal income tax purposes:
☒ Has Not Changed During Preceding 12 Months
☐ Has Changed During Preceding 12 Months (Publisher must submit explanation of change with this statement)

PS Form **3526**, July 2014 (Page 1 of 4 (see instructions page 4)) PSN: 7530-01-000-9931   PRIVACY NOTICE: See our privacy policy on www.usps.com.

13. Publication Title	14. Issue Date for Circulation Data Below
CLINICS IN PODIATRIC MEDICINE & SURGERY	JULY 2020

15. Extent and Nature of Circulation			Average No. Copies Each Issue During Preceding 12 Months	No. Copies of Single Issue Published Nearest to Filing Date
a. Total Number of Copies (Net press run)			163	149
b. Paid Circulation (By Mail and Outside the Mail)	(1)	Mailed Outside-County Paid Subscriptions Stated on PS Form 3541 (Include paid distribution above nominal rate, advertiser's proof copies, and exchange copies)	100	91
	(2)	Mailed In-County Paid Subscriptions Stated on PS Form 3541 (Include paid distribution above nominal rate, advertiser's proof copies, and exchange copies)	0	0
	(3)	Paid Distribution Outside the Mails Including Sales Through Dealers and Carriers, Street Vendors, Counter Sales, and Other Paid Distribution Outside USPS®	13	11
	(4)	Paid Distribution by Other Classes of Mail Through the USPS (e.g., First-Class Mail®)	0	0
c. Total Paid Distribution (Sum of 15b (1), (2), (3), and (4))		▶	113	102
d. Free or Nominal Rate Distribution (By Mail and Outside the Mail)	(1)	Free or Nominal Rate Outside-County Copies included on PS Form 3541	34	31
	(2)	Free or Nominal Rate In-County Copies included on PS Form 3541	0	0
	(3)	Free or Nominal Rate Copies Mailed at Other Classes Through the USPS (e.g., First-Class Mail)	0	0
	(4)	Free or Nominal Rate Distribution Outside the Mail (Carriers or other means)	0	0
e. Total Free or Nominal Rate Distribution (Sum of 15d (1), (2), (3) and (4))		▶	34	31
f. Total Distribution (Sum of 15c and 15e)		▶	147	133
g. Copies not Distributed (See Instructions to Publishers #4 (page #3))		▶	16	16
h. Total (Sum of 15f and g)		▶	163	149
i. Percent Paid (15c divided by 15f times 100)		▶	76.87%	76.69%

* If you are claiming electronic copies, go to line 16 on page 3. If you are not claiming electronic copies, skip to line 17 on page 3.

16. Electronic Copy Circulation		Average No. Copies Each Issue During Preceding 12 Months	No. Copies of Single Issue Published Nearest to Filing Date
a. Paid Electronic Copies	▶		
b. Total Paid Print Copies (Line 15c) + Paid Electronic Copies (Line 16a)	▶		
c. Total Print Distribution (Line 15f) + Paid Electronic Copies (Line 16a)	▶		
d. Percent Paid (Both Print & Electronic Copies) (16b divided by 16c × 100)	▶		

☒ I certify that 50% of all my distributed copies (electronic and print) are paid above a nominal price.

17. Publication of Statement of Ownership
☒ If the publication is a general publication, publication of this statement is required. Will be printed in the OCTOBER 2020 issue of this publication.   ☐ Publication not required.

18. Signature and Title of Editor, Publisher, Business Manager, or Owner	Date
Malathi Samayan - Distribution Controller *Malathi Samayan*	9/18/2020

I certify that all information furnished on this form is true and complete. I understand that anyone who furnishes false or misleading information on this form or who omits material or information requested on the form may be subject to criminal sanctions (including fines and imprisonment) and/or civil sanctions (including civil penalties).

PS Form **3526**, July 2014 (Page 3 of 4)   PRIVACY NOTICE: See our privacy policy on www.usps.com

Moving?

Make sure your subscription moves with you!

To notify us of your new address, find your **Clinics Account Number** (located on your mailing label above your name), and contact customer service at:

Email: journalscustomerservice-usa@elsevier.com

800-654-2452 (subscribers in the U.S. & Canada)
314-447-8871 (subscribers outside of the U.S. & Canada)

Fax number: 314-447-8029

Elsevier Health Sciences Division
Subscription Customer Service
3251 Riverport Lane
Maryland Heights, MO 63043

*To ensure uninterrupted delivery of your subscription, please notify us at least 4 weeks in advance of move.

Printed and bound by CPI Group (UK) Ltd, Croydon, CR0 4YY

03/10/2024

01040404-0008